only fat
people skip
breakfast

only fat people skip breakfast

Get Real –
THE DIET BOOK
with a Difference

LEE JANOGLY

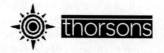

Thorsons
An Imprint of HarperCollins*Publishers*
77–85 Fulham Palace Road,
Hammersmith, London W6 8JB

The website address is: www.thorsonselement.com

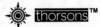

and *Thorsons* are trademarks of
HarperCollins*Publishers* Ltd

Published by Thorsons 2004

4

A catalogue record of this book is
available from the British Library

ISBN 0 00 717699 6

Printed and bound in Great Britain by
Clays Ltd, St Ives plc

In memory of my brave, beautiful friends
SHIRLEY SEGAL,
JOY STOCK
and
JILL LEVY,
who would have enjoyed this book.
I miss your laughter.

Contents

1   There Ain't No Fairy Godmother   1

2   Who's Conning Who?   27

3   The Sugar You Eat is the Fat You Wear   61

4   Your 'Living Slim' Eating Plan   97

5   You Either Get it – or You Don't   135

6   Exercise – No Sweat, No Point   172

7   You Don't Take Orders from a Biscuit   198

8   You've Lost it – Now Keep it Off Forever   246

From Me to You   287

The Binger's Psalm

On the eighth day God created cellulite.

And it came to pass that the Lord looked down upon His creation of the female form and lo, she was partaking overly of the Snickers bars and the cheese 'n' onion crisps and much of the produce of the Häagen Dazs.

And she gathered unto herself an abundance of flesh and became wide of hip and thigh and the Lord was mightily pissed off at what He saw.

So the Lord summoned his trusty prophet Bulgythias and spake unto him: 'Yo brother, dig these fat chicks! Go forth and tell 'em how it is, man.'

So the prophet Bulgythias took upon himself the task of studying the word of the diet counsellor, as it is written in the mighty tome Only Fat People Skip Breakfast *by Lee Janogly, and spake thus unto all womankind:*

'Heed my words, for if thou dost enter the portals of yonder Starbucks and order a full-fat caramel mocha latte with double cream topping, yea, verily thou shalt be great of girth and thick of thigh!

'Yield not unto temptation. Seek ye not the fruits of the sugar cane but take unto thyself the flowering broccoli instead. As thou walkest through the valley of the Marks & Spencer car park and enter the holy portals of the food hall, choose thou wisely. Gather unto thee the fish and the fowl, the fruit and the veg, and forsake all products bearing the word "frosted". Leave behind thine vehicle and power-walk around thine neighbourhood and, in time, thou shalt be rewarded with thighs that are a joy to behold – yea, a tight bum in Versace jeans shall be thine! And thine mate will be sent wild with desire, for your price is far above rubies (which doesn't say much for Ruby, but still…)

'So take heed of this wise counsel and thou shalt dwell in the House of the Slim forever. Amen.'

Telephone Conversation with a New Client (NC)

NC: *Hello? Is that the diet counsellor? I hope you can help — I'm desperate! I've got three stone to lose and it just won't shift. I've tried every diet going, but nothing works. I tried not mixing protein and carbohydrate but who can stick to that? You can't have fish and chips, there's no spag bol or burgers, so what can you eat? Then I tried that French guy's diet where you can have lots of butter and cream but that didn't work for some reason. Cabbage soup made me nauseous. As for the high-protein diet, people backed away because my breath smelt so foul and I couldn't go to the loo. But at least trying all these diets has taught me lots about nutrition. For example, I know that you must only eat fruit in the mornings because the enzyme that digests fruit doesn't work after midday...*

Me: *Oh really?*

NC: *Oh yes, didn't you know that? Anyway, so I went to Weight Watchers but I ran out of points by lunchtime. Then I did Slimming World but I accidentally had a hamburger on a green day and I'm colour-blind any- way. I couldn't work out that Zone diet, I haven't got a Little Black Dress, I read through all the blood group diets and you can eat more or less the same on all of them so what's the point? I really don't know what to do.*

Me: *Have you tried eating less?*

NC: *What do you mean?*

Chapter One

There Ain't No Fairy Godmother

I am a diet counsellor.

If you came to me for dietary advice I would assume that you wished to lose your excess weight and remain slim for the rest of your life. Obvious? Not exactly. Most people are looking for a quick fix and want instant results – and why not? That's how we approach a lot of the difficulties we encounter in our daily life, both at home and at work: identify the problem, find the solution, apply it and move on. Unfortunately, that won't work with your weight. If you've got rather more fat reserves than you need, well I bet they were there yesterday, a week ago, maybe years ago. Building them up has taken a lot of time and loving care, so it will take more than a few days of low-fat food to reduce them.

But we live in a fast-track world. Many of us are drawn to short-term, intensive deprivation diets – cabbage soup for a week, for example – in the hope of quick weight-loss, even though the weight lost on such diets is usually just water. Few people these days seem to have the patience to aim for slow, steady weight-loss that will last for life.

Many people are so eager to shed their excess pounds quickly that they become vulnerable to the allure of unhealthy or unsustainable diet regimes. There seem to be two main 'start-slimming' periods each year: the first is from the beginning of January, after the boozy excesses of Christmas, and the second starts around the end of May, with the expectation (dread?) of appearing by a pool in a bikini. In both cases, the motivation of all participants would seem to be 'How quickly can I get down to a size 10?'

Any weight you lose during this period is likely to go straight back on again. To succeed at a restrictive diet you have to ignore hunger pangs, which means you also end up ignoring feelings of satiety. Your eating 'cues' get confused and you start looking for food in response to emotional rather than physical prompts. When you follow a diet formulated by someone else, your relationship to food can be disrupted and even break down, causing you to eat in a chaotic manner.

If your most recent dieting effort ended in failure, then I'm pretty certain that the programme will have contained one of the following words or phrases: Atkins, protein-only, detox, calorie-counting, red day, points, sins, colonic, food combining, blood group, eliminate wheat/dairy/tea/coffee/alcohol. But don't despair: we've all done the same. Chalk it up to experience and now … get real!

A Long-term Approach

You don't have to be a martyr to change your lifestyle and your weight. You live in the real world where there are social occasions, celebrations, family gatherings, holidays – and supermarket checkouts stacked with chocolate bars. In this real world we experience stress, mood swings, happiness, sadness, tensions and boredom, and we are surrounded by food all the time. You need a strategy for dealing with all of this without having to think constantly 'Will I be breaking my diet?'

If you have been on the dieting seesaw for many years and know that quick-fix methods have ultimately failed you, it may now be time to take a longer-term approach – to get slim and stay slim once and for all. Then you can get on with your life.

This book contains the information you need to achieve permanent slimness. After years of diet counselling, I have realized that you can't 'treat' someone who is overweight. You can only explain the effects fat and sugar have on the body and then leave them to make their own decisions about what to eat and how much. People have to take responsibility and become self-directed.

I can only act as a guide. I will not be telling you what to eat. How can I know what you like to eat? I will advise which foods work to keep you healthy and the best time to eat them, but the final decisions are up to you. You are the one who does the eating. Only you.

🥕 **Obesity is when you weigh a stone more than your doctor.** 🥕

Get Real

It would be very easy for me to write a diet book containing 50 pages of cock-eyed theory followed by 70 pages of recipes. I am not going to do that! This is not a cookbook! There are no 'tasty recipes' – like the example I saw recently in a slimming book: 'Breakfast – a portion of smoked haddock with fine herbs, on a nest of mashed potato'. This author thinks it's feasible for you to jump out of bed, get the kids up, fed and ready for school with lunch boxes, gym clothes and homework, get yourself ready for work, then whip up a lovely dish of smoked haddock and mashed potato for breakfast. Yeah, right! Not in our world.

Every diet you have ever followed has promised that you will lose so many pounds within a certain time frame. I make no such claims because with this method you chart your own course. You will choose when to eat, what to eat and how much to eat. You will work out your own eating pattern that fits in with your lifestyle and is exclusive to you.

All you will get from me are common sense and a method that has worked for 98 per cent of my private clients (every counsellor gets one or two nutters!). If you feel that the time is right to sort out your shape once and for all, then stick around. If this is not for you, there's a whole shelf of quirky diet permutations for you to enjoy…

Let's Face It

If you're with me, we'll start with some hard facts that you may not want to hear. First, there ain't no Fairy Godmother! Sorry. No magic wands to make that fat disappear. It took time for that fat to settle so comfortably round your waist and hips – it will take time for it to go. So? What are you doing for the next few months, maybe even the next year, while you lose the weight? You will still be living the same life, with the same family, same friends, same job – only gradually getting slimmer. There's no hurry. No-one is offering you a contract to pose naked for a *Playboy* centrefold – are they?

Now the rest of the 'real deal' facts – let's get them all out of the way as quickly as possible:

1. **Your body shape is the result of your lifestyle choices.** It is the type of food you choose to eat, the quantities you serve for yourself, the exercise you do – or don't do – and the excuses you make for those decisions. All these factors determine what you look like and how you think about yourself.
2. **Losing weight starts in the mind.** If you just focus on the food, all you end up with is the Atkins Diet. The thoughts you put into your mind influence which foods

you put into your mouth. 'Ooh that looks delicious.'
'Surely a little bit won't hurt.' 'I've had a lousy week.'

If you agree with those two statements, you must also agree that the reason you are fat is because you are *choosing* to be. This is the most difficult concept to take on board, but let's face it: you are the only one who puts food in your mouth. You can't be fat unless you overeat on a regular basis, and you can't do that unless you arrange your life so that you are constantly around food. You probably use food for every occasion – as a celebration when you are happy, as a calming agent when you are stressed, as medication when you feel down, and as companionship when you feel bored or lonely.

For you, food is providing some sort of purpose other than nutrition. You are feeding some need in yourself. As long as that unacknowledged need is there, it won't make any difference which diet you follow or how many times you succeed (temporarily) in losing weight. If you don't know why you overeat, then you will never remain permanently slim.

Choosing to be Fat

Maybe you just enjoy food so much that every meal is a party and you eat more than your body needs to stay slim and healthy. Maybe you put yourself on such stringent diets that you feel deprived and end up bingeing.

Maybe you constantly tell yourself how fat and disgusting you are and how much you hate yourself, and use food to blot out the image this presents. Whatever – you are choosing to be fat.

Think carefully about this because I know your natural response will be 'How could I be *choosing* that?!' I'll tell you:

★ Every time you eat a chocolate biscuit instead of an apple, you are choosing to be fat. No, one biscuit won't make you fat but it will certainly influence what you eat later – and it reinforces that, for you, the choice is always the chocolate rather than the apple.

★ Every time you break off a chunk of cheese from a block in the fridge and pop it into your mouth, you are choosing to be fat. No, cheese is not a calcium-rich, healthy snack. It is a lump of flavoured fat – and saturated fat at that.

★ Every time you drink an extra glass of wine, which might weaken your resolve and influence your choice of food (and you know very well that it does that), you are choosing to be fat.

★ Every time you slump in front of the television on a bright, sunny evening instead of going for a walk, you are choosing to be fat.

So you see it takes quite a lot of organization to be fat. You have to actively work at it. You are not genetically programmed to carry around an excess amount of blubber, forcing your heart to work that much harder to pump blood around your body. Everyone has a natural set-point of how they are meant to look, based on their genes. Although there are some hereditary factors that will influence your shape, such as wide hipbones or thick ankles, you are not predisposed to carry vast amounts of weight around to the detriment of your health.

You can only be fat if you have created an environment that over-rides these factors and supports being overweight. Here's how to tell if you are doing it:

★ You keep a 'chocolate biscuit' cupboard in your house (for the children? Those grown-up children who left home five years ago? Or those little children who will eat whatever you give them?)
★ Your desk drawer at work resembles a sweet shop
★ You think low-fat crisps are a healthy option
★ You feel cheated if you don't have dessert in a restaurant
★ You have 'no time' for exercise
★ You get up late and have a chaotic life
★ Your social life is defined by food instead of activity
★ You are too tired after work to cook a healthy meal
★ You are contemplating taking one of those products that stops your body assimilating fat – making it OK to eat that plate of chips because the fat it contains will not be digested (dream on!)

If you keep cakes in the house, sooner or later you will eat them.

The Problems

I'm not being insensitive and certainly do not wish to discriminate against fat people – although I did have a very uncomfortable plane journey back from New York seated next to a lady who could have qualified for group medical insurance all on her own! I do know what it's like to overeat – regularly and continuously. I won't bore you – yet – with my dieting history! I do understand that whenever you overeat, you are not consciously choosing to be fat. The last thing you want to be is fat. What you are choosing is to be mindless – separating your mind from your body.

At the moment of reaching for the food you are not connecting what you are eating with the shape of your body. All you know is that you want – or *need* – to eat something, and you are choosing to ignore the fact that it will make you fat. Intellectually you know this but you are choosing to disconnect as the impulse to eat overrides the intellect. Then you profess not to understand why your excess weight won't shift.

Using Food as a Reward

Eating is a basic instinct. Scientists use mice and rats for experiments because they want to measure the results they get from basic instinct, not carefully thought-out decision-making. They program the rodents to understand that if they do what the researcher wants they will be rewarded with food. But to condition these rodents, scientists manufacture a situation where the rodents are really hungry so the food can be used as a reward. People often do the same thing to themselves to reward themselves with food. They wait until they are tired, hungry, depressed, weak, sleepy or anxious before allowing themselves to eat, then they reward themselves with fatty, sugary food.

In most aspects of your life you plan in advance: you wouldn't wait until your car was completely empty before filling it with petrol. When it comes to eating, however, many of us don't bother planning ahead. Eating can easily become something we do to respond to the moment.

Your brain naturally craves foods to meet specific needs, such as to make hormones and neurotransmitters, replace spent fuel stores or rebuild damaged muscles. By the time you crave nutrients to meet those needs, you have already suffered a deficiency. Your body signals you with urgent warnings that force you to over-correct, which means overeat. So by neglecting to feed your brain and body with what it needs before it starts a craving, you set yourself up to eat too much.

Self-esteem and Bingeing

In the fat war, there are no victims – only volunteers. That fat didn't just happen. You created the shape of your body internally, by how you feel about yourself and the things you say to yourself, and externally by the food choices you make. If you are always criticizing yourself, putting yourself down, telling yourself how awful you look, how greedy and disgusting you are, you will never lose weight permanently. No-one ever lost weight by being humiliated.

Bingers – people who use food in response to emotions rather than hunger – live with this continual low-grade preoccupation with food which erodes their self-esteem but seems normal to them. Regardless of their weight, many women feel uncomfortable about some aspect of their body. They dislike the body they live in and, as a result, end up disliking the person who lives there.

Most bingers are aware of the fact that their weight is creeping up. As weight gain is a relatively slow process, however, they tend to deny that this is happening. They refuse to admit that they eat anything fattening. 'Oh come on, a couple of biscuits at teatime isn't going to put on that much weight!' and live in a state of permanent denial. You only confront the issue when forced to do so either by a medical examination or having to let out your shower curtain! By then, instead of just dropping 10 pounds, you find you need to lose three stone to look halfway decent.

But suppose it happened overnight? Suppose you went to bed weighing 8 stone 10 and woke up the next morning weighing nearly 14 stone, fat and bloated? You would be horrified and panic-stricken, wondering what sort of disease you had contracted overnight.

The disease is eating the wrong food – that 'couple of biscuits' multiplied 20 times over, day after day, week after week. That's what you have been doing to yourself. The fact that it might have taken years rather than happened overnight is beside the point.

✸ **If the way you are behaving now is keeping you** ✸ **fat, you have to decide to behave in a different way.**

Don't be a Food Victim

It's easy to become a 'food victim' and put the blame elsewhere: your job, your mother, the kids, money problems, holidays. Sure, these can all cause stress. You can't control other people – only yourself. You can't control events – only your reaction to those events. The events will happen whether you deal with them calmly or stuff yourself with food.

You are not stupid. You know that if you eat 1,000 calories of food and only burn off 500, the other 500 are going to make their way to your fat cells and stay there. So you don't need someone to come along and tell you not to eat that extra 500 calories. Yet in spite of knowing it, you still turn to food for comfort.

And food *is* comforting. One of the first sensations

any of us can remember is being held and fed, so you equate love and food. Food is instant relief, calming, soothing your jangled nerves, banishing stress, an antidote to feeling lonely, sad, angry or depressed. So what you are doing is medicating yourself with food. You are using food to change the way you feel. As one of my diet clients explained, 'I feel as if it is the only time I can have what I want, when I want it and I don't have to explain myself to anyone.'

If you settle down in front of the television with a pile of biscuits, chocolates, crisps, fizzy drinks and ice cream, it provides instant gratification. But what you are doing is actually abusing yourself with food, the same as other people abuse alcohol or drugs. You come to rely on this type of food almost as a recreational drug to attain, fleetingly, a pleasant state of mind. By doing this you also create the need for more and more of those foods as an antidote for how they make you feel *after* the eating marathon – nauseous, bloated and dispirited about the effect on your body.

What you have to try to discover is why you are doing this. Before you start going in the right direction, you have to stop going in the wrong direction. The last thing you want is to be fat, so ask yourself if there is some aspect of your life that throws you into the kind of despair that makes you turn to food. Sometimes it can just be a stressful day, but often there may be deeper, ongoing situations that you can't change, like taking care of an elderly parent. In this case, you have to learn to deal with them without resorting to food. If you continue to binge or simply overeat regularly as your method of coping, it stops you dealing with reality. You just get instant false relief and the stressful situation remains the same.

Diet Stress

Sometimes just the thought of going on a diet – 'I'm never going to eat biscuits or cakes ever again!' – can make you feel stressed. You think of your sugar-fix as a drug and, as with any drug, you fear withdrawal symptoms or that you will feel deprived. The stress this invokes just makes you want to eat more, but this sort of stress is just something you have manufactured so that you can use it as an excuse to stuff your face.

When I ask my clients what makes them eat inappropriately, I get the following answers:

1. **Boredom.** So does eating cake relieve boredom? Boredom is a state of mind. If you are doing something that fully occupies your mind, you're not bored and don't think about eating. In truth, eating will simply intensify your boredom because the sugar makes you feel lethargic, and instead of doing some energetic physical or mental activity, you lounge around feeding your perceived feeling.
2. **It relaxes you.** Really? Yes, eating carbohydrate foods like biscuits can relieve anxiety and, as the food fills you

up, you do experience a certain relief. But what about later when you try on your favourite trousers and they won't do up? How relaxed are you then?

3. **Having a bad day.** Everyone has good and bad days, even people who don't binge. Let's face it: some days are a total waste of make-up! Eating sugary food will just make a bad day worse. You must have dealt with bad days before without bingeing, so are you just using this as an excuse to eat?

If you take the food out of the equation, you have to find another way of coping with whatever problem is driving you. Sometimes it is difficult to put your finger on exactly what is making you overeat. Maybe it started as a habit and just carried on that way. The trouble is that overeating is an auto-exacerbating disease – the more you do it, the worse it becomes. When you eat you feel guilty and disgusted with yourself, and when you feel that bad, you eat.

The only way to cure this habit is to manage it. Your eating behaviour is deeply ingrained into your subconscious. If you have binged in stressful situations in the past, you will automatically do it again, unless you can get your eating under control and change the way you think and feel about yourself. Once you admit to yourself that you do have a problem, you have taken the first step towards dealing with it.

You have coped before. You can cope again. Do not turn to food. Food will not change the situation. It will only make you feel worse.

Don't do Diets

First, though, you have to realize that no-one and no
'dietary method' can do it for you. Although most diets
don't cause eating disorders, most eating disorders begin
with a diet. Going on a diet can disrupt your physical
sense of when and how much to eat, and can lead to
bingeing. Sticking to a restricted eating plan can in itself
promote that 'Oh sod it' response of bingeing on vast
quantities of food when anything disrupts your strict
sense of being 'good'.

The typical dieter's mind-set is that if eating makes
you fat then not eating must make you slim. But trying
not to eat is not being in control because your body per-
ceives this as starvation and will set up an enormous
craving until you give in. This is simply your body's way
of making sure you stay alive.

Even on 'Eat-as-much-as-you-like' weight-loss regimes
like the high-protein Atkins diet, there are pitfalls, as
described by writer Allison Pearson in the *Evening
Standard*. She, 'like half of London', is 'doing Atkins' and
says it goes something like this: 'Atkins, Atkins, biscuit,
oops (not very Atkins), Atkins, white wine, oh God, sorry.
Atkins says eat cheese and butter, but how can you eat
cheese and butter without crackers? I am allowed to eat
double cream but no berries. Atkins, Atkins, croissant...'

Those who are not on the Atkins diet seem to be on a
'counting' diet. I have had it up to here with counting!
Everybody I meet is counting something: points, calories,
sins, fat units, stones, pounds, kilos, dress sizes, days ('I've

been good for four days now', 'I haven't had chocolate for two weeks', 'This week I've done three red days and four green days'. What *are* you going on about, woman?). Is this some sort of endless numbers game? Stop counting!

The overwhelming sense of dissatisfaction my clients express with commercial diet plans comes from the realization that they simply do not work in the long term. It's not that surprising, though. If you were a research animal, maybe a kindly scientist could deliver you precisely the amount and type of food that would achieve the weight-loss you want – and you could just lie around in a cosy cage while it happened. But you are a human being and your life is not lived in a laboratory.

You probably already know from bitter experience that following a particular diet theory may produce startling weight-loss results while you stick to it. But if, in a year's time, you are back where you started, was it worth it? And once you climb on the dieting seesaw, it is very difficult to get off. The diet habit becomes deeply ingrained as a way of life and the 'language' is imprinted on your brain.

You are always thinking about food, evaluating the calorie content, having those 'Shall I, shan't I?' conversations in your head about some fattening item of food, usually ending with 'Oh well, I've blown it now. I might as well go on eating for the rest of the day and start my diet again tomorrow'.

Bear this in mind: **dieters always eat much more when they think they have 'broken their diet' than**

people who never diet at all. The urge is to cram it all in now so they can start tomorrow with a clean slate (plate?). The only way to stop this is to get off it. Lose the dieting mentality. If you want to be permanently slim, you have to change the way you think, act and behave.

It is no accident that some people are fat. This is a disease of choice. People carrying a lot of extra weight may have a slower metabolism but they are still making choices. You can either choose to eat something fattening or choose to eat something non-fattening. Maybe you choose the fattening option every time? If so, why? You have to acknowledge that if you choose to behave in a certain way, you also choose the results of that behaviour. It may not be ideal but it's the only deal you've got. There is no point in saying 'I'm going to do this or that' – you have to *activate* the plan and start doing something.

The Solution

Be Accountable

Acknowledge and accept accountability for the shape of your body. You are accountable for the type of food you put into your mouth – not some of the time but all of the time. If you follow someone else's diet that tells you what to eat at each meal, you are simply handing over your responsibility. When you don't lose weight, it is the 'diet' that didn't work, thereby absolving you of all blame.

You are accountable for the way you see yourself and

the way you feel. If, at times, you are angry, hurt or upset, then *those are your feelings* and you are accountable for their presence in your life. Whatever your circumstances, accepting this key premise – whether you like it or not – means you can no longer dodge responsibility for the position you find yourself in.

If you think I'm labouring this point – I am! If you don't accept accountability, if you insist that you 'can't help' being overweight, nothing will ever change, plain and simple. By convincing yourself that you are a victim and 'can't stop eating' (of course you can), that you 'really try' (obviously not hard enough) and that you 'hardly eat anything' (who are you kidding?), you will stay stuck on the diet/binge seesaw for the foreseeable future.

The only person you can rely on to change your life is *you*. You have free choice. You make the decisions about what you are going to eat; you take responsibility for your shape, your health, your level of fitness and the thoughts that govern all of the above. Once you acknowledge that you are in charge of your life and your eating, it will happen.

🌀 **Self-choice isn't deprivation – it's freedom.** 🌀

Get Positive

To get a clearer picture of how things will be, you have to move towards something positive, not just away from something negative. Create a picture in your mind: in this corner there is 'you' – overweight, feeling heavy and lumpy and hating yourself. This is a very painful state to be in. Over in that corner is 'you' as you want to be – slim, light and attractive and feeling good about yourself. No pain there. When you have embarked on a weight-loss programme before, you have simply gone on a restrictive diet without a clear plan or strategy. At the beginning, your motivation is obviously high. As the pounds disappear you begin to move away from the 'fat you' corner and the pain lessens slightly. Then when the hunger and cravings start to kick in, you go back to your old habits and begin to eat a 'little bit' of the fattening foods you ate before. Soon you get sucked back into the fat corner because nothing has really changed. You have simply gone on a diet without changing your behaviour or your lifestyle, without including any extra activity into your life, without a specific strategy for change.

If you keep on doing the same, you will keep on getting the same. However, once you stop being reactive and make a definite commitment to change your way of life, you will gradually and steadily start to move towards the positive corner, and become the slim 'you' that you want to be. In this way, you are not just moving away from something negative – the 'fat you' – but *towards* something positive – the 'slim you'.

To do this you have to be very clear about how your life will be different once you have lost the excess weight. What aspects of your life would you have to overcome or change in order to become the person you want to be? What are you doing right now – or not doing – to impede your efforts to get slim?

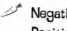 **Negative thoughts produce negative results.**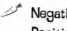
Positive thoughts produce positive results.

Be Mentally Slim

To be a slim person, you have to live like a slim person. You have to *see* yourself as a slim person. This means having a very clear picture in your mind of what it is like to *be* a slim person, how to *behave* like a slim person, how to *present* yourself as a slim person, all the time. You have to mentally *turn into* that person. Even though you are not there yet, by pretending that you are, by *acting* as though the weight has already gone, you are programming yourself to succeed.

A slim person is not someone who is on a diet. She does not wake up and tell herself that she will be 'good' today. Acting slim means that when you look in the mirror you don't dwell on the rolls of fat round your waist and hips. You simply check that the clothes you are wearing look OK and move on. It means you don't call yourself names like 'greedy pig' and tell yourself you look 'fat and revolting'.

Slim people see themselves as attractive and energetic. They automatically veer towards healthy food and limit their intake of the more fattening varieties. They would rather eat two squares of good quality chocolate than gorge on several bars of the cheaper kind.

Slim people do not have a problem making food choices. They do not agonize over whether they should or shouldn't eat some fattening item of food in case it starts them eating for the rest of the day. They simply avoid eating obviously fattening food because they know it will make them fat. Fat people know this too but always seem to be amazed and depressed when it happens.

The rules for living like a slim person are very simple:

★ You have to be in control of your eating – no mindless picking.

★ You have to make a commitment to eat healthy food. If you want to be slim there is no point eating the sort of food that makes you fat. This food usually contains refined sugar.

★ You have to delete the diet mentality – whether you are having a 'good' or a 'bad' day, meaning whether or not you ate anything fattening today.

★ You have to change the way you behave. If your life is one chaotic rush with no time for anything, that has to be sorted.

★ You have to make time for some regular activity in your life. Everyone can find 20 minutes a day for exercise if they want to.

★ You have to change the way you think about yourself and the way you think about food.

★ Most importantly, you need to have a clear picture in your head of what you want to look like when you have lost your excess weight, what you will *feel* like when you are slim, how you will *behave* when you are slim.

Once you know what you really want – a slim, healthy body – getting there takes resolve and commitment. If you have spent most of your life just moaning about what you *don't want* – how you hate being fat, how you can't stop eating – then simply making the commitment to be slim will seem unnatural.

⊛   **Lose the 'fat' thoughts in your head and you**   ⊛
will lose the fat on your thighs.

Stop Lying

All bingers lie – to themselves and to others. Seventeen-stone clients swear to me that nothing passes their lips except lettuce and cottage cheese. Come on now, you *know* biscuits make you fat and you also know that one biscuit won't do that. But taking the view that 'one biscuit won't make a difference' leads to 'just a few nuts/an ice cream/one slice of pizza/two squares of chocolate – won't make a difference'. Individually, maybe not – if you are already slim. But collectively, every day, they do. So why are you surprised when this happens?

'I'll start again tomorrow.' Why? What makes you think it will be easier tomorrow, especially if you are planning to activate your sugar-craving with an almighty binge for the rest of the day? Stop kidding yourself. Are you going to wait until you are another stone heavier before you start doing something about it? There is only one life; this is not a dress rehearsal for the slim life you should be living. Only you can bring that about.

As Professor Ben Fletcher of the Framework of Internal Transformation (FIT) says: 'You get what you expect. If you are not getting what you want, you have to change your thinking slightly. Because we are such habitual creatures, we cocoon ourselves in the world that we had yesterday. We like the comfort of what we know. People have the illusion that they are flexible, and this is especially true of leaders, politicians and chief executives. In fact, many are prisoners of their habits.'

The simple, obvious premise outlined in the following pages will give you the knowledge and tools to change the habits that have kept you fat. It will enable you to live the rest of your life as a slim person. You can choose to use these tools at any time. Sometimes you may disregard them and put on a few pounds, but once this knowledge is firmly implanted in your head, you can use it to get back on track any time you choose.

♂ **Whether you believe you can or you believe** ♂
you can't, you're right!

Conversation with Client

C: *Will you just verify something for me: my hairdresser says that you need four tablespoons of olive oil every day to keep your hair strong and shiny and that a low-fat diet will cause dryness of the hair and scalp.*

Me: *I don't think your hairdresser knows what he's talking about. Even if you cut down drastically on your fat consumption, if you are eating a balanced diet you will still be getting more fat than you need to keep everything properly lubricated, including your hair and scalp.*

C: *Oh. He also says that to lose weight you should eat half a grapefruit before each meal. How does that work?*

Me: *It doesn't – unless you don't actually eat the meal after you've had the grapefruit! Which I don't advise, by the way. What other gems does this font of all nutritional knowledge have to impart?*

C: *Well, apparently, to speed up weight loss you should eat negative-value foods like celery and radishes. He says this sort of food burns up more calories in the chewing and digesting than is actually contained in the food.*

Me: *That's a load of rubbish. What else?*

C: *Come on, he's really knowledgeable. Did you know that to make your nails grow stronger you should eat jelly or dip your hands in it because it contains gelatin?*

Me: *Well, if you want to sit with your hand in a bowl of jelly, then don't let me stop you. Which nutritional academy did this genius graduate from?*

C: *The Morris School of Hairdressing.*

Me: *I thought so.*

C: *You are being very unkind. He knows a lot about nutrition. He told me that pineapples contain a special enzyme that burns up fat. Is that true?*

Me: *Wrong again. Pineapples do contain an enzyme called bromelin, which digests protein and is similar to an enzyme called papain in papayas. These are not found in any other fruits but, sadly, they do not burn up fat. There is no food yet invented that does. Even if there were, you wouldn't be able to find it because I would have bought up the entire supply!*

C: *But surely he is right about some things?*

Me: *Well, he has cut one side of your hair shorter than the other. That should tell you something.*

Chapter Two

Who's Conning Who?

'In the year 500 BC (Before Conley – of the Sainted Rosemary), the Prophet Legawaxius declared (from the Book of Salon, App. 10.30, Bikini-Line 1): "If thou dost prevail and surrender thine body into the hands of practitioners well versed in the art of beautifying the flesh, be it encumbered upon you to preserve thy maidenly modesty by remaining clothed in thy garment of knicker – be it elephantipants or thong – at all times."'

How the Diet Industry Gets Rich

As a dieter you are part of a very exploited group. An £80 million diet industry thrives on your failure. To the pharmaceutical industry, fat people represent a potentially unrivalled source of revenue. Having found a cure for impotence with Viagra, it now sees a remedy for obesity as its holy grail. Even the reputable slimming organizations would surely prefer that you fail so that you will keep coming back and paying your weekly dues. How else can they make money?

Slimming Aids

The same applies to the slimming aids you can buy over-the-counter in chemist or health-food shops. People keep buying these products then blaming themselves when they don't work. The diet companies are making a fortune persuading you to buy these pills or food substitutes on the assumption that they will make you feel and look better. But do they? You tell me.

While there are reputable manufacturers of diet products, there is also a huge market in what can only be described as weight-loss fraud. As long as people are prepared to try to lose weight at any cost there will continue to be 'entrepreneurs' who exploit that desire by selling bogus products.

Recently I received an 'invitation' through the post to buy an 'all natural' tablet whose main unspecified ingredient reportedly helped dieters lose 72 pounds in 10 weeks – a result, which I imagine, could be achieved only by amputation. If I sent off my application 'immediately' I would be lucky enough to get an extra week's supply of these fabulous capsules absolutely free. I can't wait!

According to the product blurb, if I take just two tablets each day I will lose as much weight as I want and – yippee! – my metabolism will increase to such an extent that the fat will drop off my body (into a greasy puddle on the floor?). Developed in Switzerland (why is that meant to impress?) by doctors (not window cleaners then?), these tablets mean I will never feel hungry. Amazingly, I will never have to diet again as the tablets will be 'retraining my body's ability to convert fat to energy'. Thank goodness for that then.

The leaflet accompanying this miraculous, 100-percent herbal fat-burner shows a studious-looking man in a white coat wielding a stethoscope (in case I didn't believe the 'doctor' bit?). The wording is full of scientific terms that seem to suggest the product has been created as a result of exciting new research into lipogenesis – the metabolic processes by which fat is stored in the body. The unique ingredient (still unnamed) is 'especially relevant for people whose calorie consumption exceeds healthful levels'.

These claims are designed to persuade you that if a product is 'relevant' to overeating, you will stay fat forever if you don't use it. The fear factor! Are you convinced?

If you're looking for a quick-fix slimming aid, you are undoubtedly well served by manufacturers of diet products. It is a terrific industry – I wish I'd thought of it! But do we really believe we can buy a product and it will make us slimmer? Aren't we just buying a fantasy? Some people buy Lottery tickets and dream about becoming a millionaire. Others buy diet products and dream of becoming slim. It's the same thing (except that there's a very small chance of actually winning the Lottery).

If there were indeed a safe, authorized, over-the-counter product that could make a fat person slim, we would all know about it. We would have read about it in a respected medical journal. There would have been controlled medical tests, serious long-term research and all the endorsements in place from government drug-safety administrations to license the product for sale. More to the point, everyone who wanted to be slim would be. But they aren't. So that magic product or ingredient isn't available. This doesn't stop manufacturers claiming their diet products achieve this effect or, if they're more responsible, suggesting that they can help you lose weight as part of a properly managed diet plan.

Sometimes these products are endorsed by doctors, who extol the safety and benefits of the tablets, potions or supplements. Personally, I believe that any doctors endorsing a diet product should be made to declare whether they have a financial interest in that product or are being paid any kind of commission.

Any product that promises instant success without the chore of dieting and exercise is a real concern to me. Such claims simply divert consumers from considering healthier ways of controlling their weight. Moreover, there can be serious side-effects from taking more than the recommended dose on the packet, and many dieters do this, as the diet mentality dictates that if one tablet or tea bag will make you slim, then five will make you slimmer.

In an image-obsessed culture, where companies market diet products aggressively to exploit people's dissatisfaction with their looks, common sense sometimes loses out. Even though, intellectually, many people know the products won't work, their desire to lose weight – to find a short cut so that they can be accepted, admired and successful – is so strong that it's worth £29.99 just to buy into the fantasy.

     Stop deluding yourself. You can't have it all.
     You can try. You have tried. It doesn't work.

Creaming off the Profits

Talking of cost, hands up who has paid a large amount
of dosh for a cream that you rub in your thighs and bottom to get rid of cellulite? Oh, come on, you haven't!
And did it work? Did it get rid of the fat? Where did
the fat go – to your stomach, your ankles, the bloodstream? If you had a bath in the cream, would you
emerge slimmer all over?

A marketing friend told me about a campaign that
was initiated to create massive demand for a cream that
would reduce fat on the thighs. The plan was to create a
huge buzz about the product before it was launched –
and it worked magnificently. It was so simple: just a little whisper in a few susceptible ears: 'It's only available in
France at the moment!', 'They're queuing round the
block to get it', 'It's selling out over there', 'Coming here
soon!', 'Really expensive!', 'Limited stocks when it does
arrive', 'Quick – before they sell out!'.

And the inevitable result? 'How do I get it?', 'Where
can I get it?' Rather ordinary smoothing cream becomes
the must-have new product before it is even packaged in
the expensively designed pot, because no-one wants to
be the only person left in town with fat thighs.

Don't worry. You didn't miss anything. As one doctor
said, 'If this cream has any effect on physiological function,

then legally it should be sold as a drug. If it doesn't have any effect, why should anyone buy it?'

For the sake of your body and your bank balance, understand this: you cannot break down fat from the outside. The only way fat gets on your body is when you eat more food than you expend in energy, and the excess gets stored in your cells. Therefore the only way to get rid of it is to make sure it gets used up as energy – and you know exactly how that works. A cream that could dissolve fat would have to dissolve the skin first – think about it!

There is a discrepancy between the manufacturers' and the public's perception of what constitutes a 'cure' for cellulite, or cauliflower bottom syndrome (CBS). The manufacturers assume it is to make the skin smoother and less lumpy-looking; the user wants to end up two inches slimmer.

Beware Beauty Salon Treatments

Save your money. Any treatment undertaken in a beauty salon which claims to make you slimmer by applying ointment, clay, slimy gunge, or attacking your thighs with nasty-looking instruments, tight bandages (to squish the fat into submission?), electrical impulse treatment, or whatever, is a complete waste of time. Little electrical impulses to stimulate your muscles will have no impact on the surrounding fat. Similarly, there is no such thing as a 'non-invasive' face-lift.

You should also be wary of suggestions made by the attractive, slim beauty therapist attending to your vulnerable thighs while you lie prone in your cubicle. A white nylon coat and a name tag do not confer instant qualifications upon the wearer. The letters after her name are probably her postcode.

Aspiring beauty therapists are indoctrinated with three key phrases: 'Breaks down the fat', 'Increases the circulation' and 'Gets rid of toxins' (sound familiar?). Therapists are instructed to repeat these phrases at intervals during each consultation with a client, in the firm belief that said client will not dispute this. Asking for a more detailed analysis, 'What do you mean it breaks down the fat?' will elicit the response, 'You know, it breaks down the fat so that it can be carried away by your increased circulation'. Don't bother to ask 'How?' or 'Where does it get carried to?' – she doesn't know and you will only confuse her.

You will certainly be lighter when you leave the beauty salon – by at least 50 or 60 pounds – but only in your wallet. And news travels fast, so if by the remotest chance any of these anti-fat treatments worked then nobody would have any fat. Surely this should tell you something. However, there's no telling some people – and with time on your hands, fat on your thighs and money in your pocket, the choice is yours.

You could even join Cherie Blair on her Detox Slimming Machine. Appearing svelte and slim(ish) at the Labour Party Conference in October 2003, the prime minister's wife was reportedly very enthusiastic about her three-times-a-week slimming treatments to get rid of 'toxic waste' and reverse years of 'digestive abuse'. The treatment consists of lying on a couch and being attached to 32 electrodes that emit electrical currents to tap away at the 'intestinal plaque' lining the colon and intestines. A course of 12 sessions costs £695. A laxative would have the same effect at a fraction of the price as would taking a natural product like psysllium or ispaghula husk, marketed in the UK as Fybogel. You are also advised to go on a strict detoxification diet – eating only fruit, vegetable soup and salad with a small meal of chicken and rice for dinner. Oh really? No sausage, bacon and chips then?

Let's talk toxins for a moment. A toxin is a poison usually produced in the body by bacteria. *Health Encyclopaedia*, the medical guide used by the Royal Society of Medicine, suggests that bacterial toxins are extremely dangerous, and if they enter the blood in more than minute quantities, the effects are always serious. If you suffered the build-up of toxins suggested by these so-called 'health experts' you would probably be dead, and the idea that you can be 'cured' of toxins by electrical stimulation, colonic irrigation or a detox diet is ludicrous. **Not one toxin, as the term is understood by the Royal Society of Medicine, can be removed by any detox programme.**

As Amanda Wynne, a spokesperson for the British Dietetic Association tactfully put it: 'I can't really comment on this so-called detoxifying process but the diet doesn't sound hugely nutritious to me. You can lose between one and two pounds a week quite easily just by eating healthily and exercising – and save yourself £695.'

If you have that much money to spare, why not go for surgery? Plastic surgeons have developed a technique to get rid of the 'orange peel' effect of cellulite by snipping the ligaments just under the skin to produce a smoother look (Tucks R Us?). Unfortunately, this doesn't eliminate the fat; you just look smooth and fat instead of lumpy and fat. Fatso intacto.

The only plastic surgery that will effectively protect you from all of the above is to cut up your credit cards.

Fad Diets

Even if you don't succumb to slimming treatments, nothing it seems will deter you from going on your next diet. Over the years the professional dieter must have lost at least 40 stone. Each new diet promises you more food than you can eat, instant results and strangers on the bus coming up and asking you to dance.

Let's face it: authors write diet books to make money. If they can think up some weird food permutation – the quirkier the better – that captures the public imagination, they are laughing. Even better, if loads of people try it and lose weight – as you do – word of mouth is the best publicity. What doesn't concern these writers, however, is the effects their methods could have on someone's health if they stay on the diet for a long period.

🥕 **If you keep repeating the same action, you** 🥕
will keep getting the same results.

High-protein, Low-carb Regimes

In the same week it was announced that the Atkins diet book – which advocates foods high in protein and fat and low in carbohydrates – was rivalling Harry Potter in sales, a report was published in the *Lancet* medical journal linking too much fatty food with an increased risk of breast cancer.

Dr Sheila Bingham, who led the study for the European Prospective Investigation of Cancer and Nutrition said: 'The effect seems to be related particularly to saturated fat found mostly in butter, meat, lamb, sausages, bacon and cheese,' foods which are the main staples of the Atkins diet. Women eating the most fat had a 33 per cent extra risk of developing the disease.

So – are you dying to be slim?

Another report by Dr Bill Robertson, a clinical biochemist at the Institute of Urology at the University College Medical School, claims that although you could lose a stone on the Atkins diet, you could also gain a stone – in your kidney. Kidney stones are extremely painful hard deposits that often need an operation or laser treatment to remove them. Dr Robertson says, 'It (The Atkins Diet) is the worst possible combination. The absence of fruit and vegetables means the body is deprived of a means of counteracting the negative effect of a diet rich in animal proteins and calcium oxalate. The high-protein diets have contributed to an increase in the number of kidney stones that we are seeing.'

Are you suffering to be slim?

These reports have caused the Atkins company to hastily 'revise' how the diet should be used. It appears the consumer 'misunderstood' Dr Atkins' use of the phrase 'eat liberally' in relation to foods high in saturated fat, and are now advised to place more emphasis on fish and chicken rather than red meat. In other words, 'Please don't sue us if you get sick.'

Television personality, Anne Diamond, now more well-known for her fluctuating body shape than her presenting skills, described being on the Atkins diet as follows: 'In my view, the Atkins diet is a recipe for a revolting feeling of bloated over-consumption, coupled with a disgusting, fatty taste in your mouth and breath like vapours from a compost heap. I tried it for six days. In the end, I gave up because I felt so nauseous, and I was seriously worried about my heart.'

Anne finally went to her GP with palpitations. Once he knew what she had been eating, he said, 'Stop being so bloody silly and to go back to eating proper food in moderation.' That'll learn yer!

In the short term, a high-protein diet does little harm. The trouble is, it just encourages yo-yo dieting where you lose significant amounts of weight quickly, and put it back on as soon as you start eating 'normally' – then you have to go on the diet again to lose it, and so on. According to doctors, this sort of fluctuation is more dangerous than staying permanently at a slightly inflated weight.

An interesting fact to emerge from the Atkins diet is that, contrary to previous thinking about weight, dietary fat doesn't make you fat – in fact, in the absence of carbohydrates it appears to have the opposite effect, albeit only while you adhere to this formula. It is *sugar* that makes you fat, and the fat/sugar combo found in cakes, biscuits and the like is the surest way to increase your girth.

So Why Diet?

The stupid thing is that most dieters are not significantly overweight. Dieting has become so much part of our culture that many people, especially women, go on diets regardless of their actual weight on the assumption that, no matter what they weigh, it would be better to weigh less.

  ♂ **The 'what should be' never did exist but people** ♂
     keep trying to live up to it. There is no
     'what should be' – there is only what is.

Social Conditioning

Women are particularly vulnerable to the diet-based lifestyle. Girls tend to learn from an early age that their worth can be measured on a set of bathroom scales, and it sets the pattern for a lifetime of dissatisfaction with how they look. A study carried out by the University of London in September 2003 involving nearly 3,000 youngsters from 28 schools, found that almost half of the girls aged 11 to 14 were trying to lose weight. Most modelled themselves on Victoria Beckham and admitted to skipping meals in their efforts to adhere to the latest manifestation of a world gone mad, where women are supposed to look like pre-pubescent boys with big tits. By the time these girls become young adults, they will have internalized the belief that there is something wrong with them for being their natural size or slightly bigger. They think it is their fault and collude with the culture that tells them they should be thin to be worthwhile.

Guilt

This is why all dieters feel guilty about eating – whatever they eat. Even though they enjoy the taste of food, they usually gulp it down quickly. This is because, subconsciously, they feel they are doing something wrong by eating anything at all – although logically they know they have to eat to stay alive.

Guilt is also the reason they put themselves on horrendous detox regimes, living on just fruit juice for a week with all the discomfort, headaches, weakness and coated tongue that are the inevitable results. And when they feel that bad they think they deserve it because this is the price for eating too much and becoming fat.

People go on strict diets to punish themselves for being fat – for overeating.

Once you understand that diets are punishments for bad behaviour, you can understand why they fail. Eating is not a crime but you behave as though it were. Diets are like being in prison where you do 'time' for not looking right: 'I've done three days now'. Prisoners, however, become rebellious. Regardless of how willingly you entered your diet-cell, after a while you begin to think about breaking out. Convicts fantasize about a cake with a file in it. Dieters just fantasize about the cake.

A Distorted Self-image

Most dieters have such a distorted view of their own bodies that they don't know what their genetic shape should be. They accept the idea that there is an 'ideal' body and that theirs is far from it. So whenever they feel bad about themselves, regardless of the cause, they say they 'feel fat'.

Although you see yourself as weak-willed, self-indulgent and lacking in self-discipline, none of this is true. No-one has ever tried more diligently to solve a problem than the chronic dieter. You have followed every recommendation ever made regarding the best way to approach what you see as your problem. You have deprived yourself of food in endless ways, and spent time, energy and money in your efforts to find the answer.

Unfortunately, the diets you have embarked upon have always failed you in some way because, if you are an over-eater or binger, once that urge to eat is upon you, there is no way you could stick to a diet devised by someone else. These diets never address your need to turn to food when under stress. That is why only four dieters out of every hundred keep the weight off.

Even now, scientists are testing production of a new, 'safer' diet pill – one that will eliminate hunger without the damaging side-effects of previously used amphetamine-based drugs. They might as well not bother. Most overweight women do not eat because they are hungry. They eat because they are tense, stressed, bored and often because they are depressed at being fat. How many times has the following scenario been played out by a woman and her concerned partner:

Him: *Why are you eating that?*
Her: *Because I'm fat.*
Him: *But if you finish that whole packet you'll be even fatter.*
Her: *I know. I don't care.*
Him: *But you do care. You keep saying how miserable you are because you're fat.*
Her: *Just LEAVE IT will you! I'll do it when I'm ready.*

That's it, mister, leave it. She *will* do it but in her own time. Any word from you will send her diving into the biscuit tin.

You may not believe it, but you are not deliberately being self-destructive if you eat when you're not hungry. You eat at these times because it feels 'right' to you

– as if food will 'help'. And you'd be right. For many years, compulsive eating has provided you with a coping mechanism.

So it makes no sense to assume that the thousands of people who are currently dieting are somehow deficient, that they lack the strength of character to achieve anything, particularly when many of them succeed in their pursuit of goals in other areas of their lives. Those shapeless women Members of Parliament who reach the front benches and look as if they get dressed in the dark are a good example. Clearly there must be something in every diet that ensures its ultimate failure, regardless of how long it's been in the bestseller list.

Dieters always assume every aspect of their lives will be perfect in a smaller size. They cling to the belief that the next diet will be their passport to a better life, and they are putting everything on hold until this magic moment arrives. Compulsive eaters can't imagine not being on a diet – the only alternative lifestyle they see involves eating everything in sight.

The truth is that if people ate natural produce all the time, including grains, fish, chicken, fruit and vegetables – even a certain amount of butter or oil – they would be slim and have adequate nutrition. Highly processed, fatty, artificially sweetened stuff just confuses your system. Your body simply doesn't know what to do with the chemicals. Ultimately, this sort of food is not satisfying so you crave more of it, and you lose track of the brain's usual regulatory signals that tell you whether you are hungry or full up. When your body doesn't get what it wants, it keeps trying, eating till it is satisfied.

As a seasoned dieter, you probably welcome the rules and regulations of a new diet and feel relief to be able to hand over your food decisions to the author, assuming they must know what they are talking about. But diets never live up to their promises if they prescribe some quirky food permutation or are very restrictive. You will always find a reason to go back to what you consider to be 'normal eating'.

Media Pressure

The media doesn't help. Editors of women's magazines are constantly under pressure to come up with news about dieting to feed their readers' presumably insatiable desires for weight-loss advice. Although some of these magazines are cautious and thorough in their approach to nutrition reporting, a 'diet breakthrough' is just too hard to resist writing about – as the editors will tell you, they have to give the readers what they want!

You will have seen countless articles in magazines saying 'Diets Don't Work' followed, 20 pages later, by a 'Get Slim for Summer' feature. Everyone who reads the message that diets don't work resists it. You cling to the belief that you *can* find a way to make one work. Look at all those 'before' and 'after' pictures of people who have tried to lose weight for those beach photos. Surely if it works for them it will work for you. (Secret: what the magazine didn't tell you is that the people in the 'after' pictures didn't make it through to 'Still Slim in Spring', and neither will you.)

Some writers are paid by product companies to place promotional articles in magazines. The pressure on editors to fill their magazine content every month with new stories can lead to reporters and feature writers falling back on 'press-release journalism', which means they will simply reproduce material sent to them by PR companies – and every magazine editor is bombarded with press releases all the time eulogizing new products and services for their readers.

The press release may sound scientific, or may even be issued from a reputable university or research institute. The 'experts' quoted, however, may have some financial interest in the product they are promoting, or might even influence the editor by placing a full-page advert for the product in the magazine.

To enhance readers' interest, the magazine will list famous people who apparently swear by the stuff. In recent years it must seem as though Geri Halliwell, Liz Hurley and Madonna are the recipients of every weight-loss and beauty aid invented!

What about adverts you see or hear on radio or television? How objective are they? When food manufacturers sponsor television programmes, how much could they, or do they, influence the content of that programme? Do we even think about it when we see the logos come up and hear 'this programme is brought to you by' or 'in association with'? In one country, a well-known fast-food manufacturer even sponsors the news bulletins on one channel. Now how much critical comment are you going to get about junk food from that television station?

Newspapers and magazine editors and makers of lifestyle programmes for radio and television know that dieters love to hear the latest scientific discoveries. This audience, however, is not looking for the latest news about a cure for cancer; they just want to read that someone has invented a lettuce that tastes of chocolate. Editors and programme-makers therefore owe it to all of us to ensure that their stories about 'diet breakthroughs' are informed with broad research and deep scepticism – but don't hold your breath for that.

The Triumph of Hope over Experience

You would think that people who have spent their adult years failing at diets would be relieved to discover that they don't have to try every new one that comes out. But that's not the case. If there is the slightest suggestion that they might be able to 'Get Slim for Summer', they want to give it a try.

Professor Janet Polivy, from the psychology department at the University of Toronto, conducted some very interesting research studies a few years ago. She found that simply going on a diet disrupted people's physical sense of when and how much to eat – and this led to overeating. In experiments where dieters had to eat a high-calorie snack, thereby purposely breaking their diet, they ate much more than non-dieters in the same situation. Furthermore, they ate more than non-dieters when they *believed* the snack was high-calorie, even when it was in fact low-calorie.

In tests where dieters thought they were being watched after breaking their diet, they ate very little; but afterwards, when they thought they were alone, they would binge. Again and again the researchers provided evidence for what they came to call the 'what-the-hell' effect of overeating after breaking a diet – and what I call the 'Oh sod it!' syndrome.

Every time you put yourself on a strict diet you are trying to train yourself to give precedence to what the diet allows over what the body demands. That would be fine if the body demanded only what the diet allowed but this is rarely the case. The crucial problem with all restrictive dieting is that it drives a wedge between the person and her body; a struggle ensues and generally the situation deteriorates until the dieter has wrecked the natural signals, since these signals are what the diet is designed to override.

So out goes eating on the basis of natural hunger cues and in come calorie calculations or peculiar nutritional combinations, in particular the current fashion of cutting out entire food groups such as wheat, dairy, tea, coffee, sugar and alcohol. This leads to emotional bingeing and being controlled by the vast swathes of foods you are try-ing to eliminate.

This turns you into a binger, eating on the basis of compulsion, obeying mysterious urges to eat that correspond neither to the original hunger that is entirely natural nor even to the diet that you substituted for natural eating.

✐ 'Low-fat' doesn't mean 'not fattening' if you ✐
eat a lot of it.

The Binger

Let's profile the binger for a moment. Not all dieters are bingers. Some people are overweight because they just eat too much of the wrong foods at mealtimes and do no exercise. Bingers are another category altogether and comprise a significant proportion of my clients.

Compulsive eating is more than an activity; it is an all-absorbing state of mind. Bingers come in all shapes and sizes and lead all kinds of emotional lives. What they share is their obsession with food and weight. This dual preoccupation with food and body shape is the hallmark of the compulsive eater.

The clients who consult me are not necessarily very fat. Although we are accustomed to equating fat with gluttony, I have found that the shape of someone's body is not necessarily a reliable indicator of their relationship with food. Some people come to me just to learn how to stop bingeing. Although their weight fluctuates wildly over a six-month period, they don't allow a binge to go on long enough to cause a lasting weight increase. They go back to a strict diet to bring it down again. As one of them said, 'No-one believes me when I say I have an eating problem. I know I don't look as though I have, but not a day goes by when I don't obsess about food.' Privately, I call these 'thin fat people'.

Most bingers though, offer convincing proof of their struggle by their increased girth. They are constantly eating more food than their bodies require, reaching for food for emotional reasons rather than natural hunger, and if they do start out hungry, they continue to eat way past the point of physiological satiation. Therefore, no-one can diagnose compulsive eating based on size. Only you know if you are a binger.

Given the all-too-human capacity for denial, a binger is simply unaware of the inordinate amount of time she spends thinking about, choosing, buying, cooking and eating food. (I use the term 'she' because most bingers are women but that's not to ignore those many men who have the problem.)

For our typical binger, her mealtimes, socializing, weekends and celebrations are the focus of her food obsession: what she should or shouldn't be eating, will she manage to stick to her diet, is she having a 'good' day? So much mental energy is expended on a substance she is trying desperately not to eat.

It is senseless to label a binge habit simply as obesity – just as you can't say that alcoholism is simply drunkenness or drug addiction merely the problem of being stoned. The fat is simply the symptom of the underlying eating disorder, albeit a significant one.

Most bingeing is done in the hours between the evening meal and bedtime – unless you are a mum with young children, when it starts at afternoon teatime. Food eaten during the early part of the day doesn't seem to stimulate the need to continue eating as much as the evening meal does – probably because most people's days are fairly structured and food eaten towards the end of the day signals a release of tension.

There is a difference between the eating habits of an 'overeater' and a 'binger'. Returning from work, an overeater will nibble on peanuts or olives with her alcoholic drink while preparing the evening meal. This will probably consist of something like thick soup with a roll and butter, followed by roast beef, Yorkshire pudding, roast potatoes, rice and a green vegetable. She will finish with apple pie and custard or ice cream. Tea and cake will follow a couple of hours later. She can't understand why eating this way – plus a substantial breakfast and lunch – keeps her fat.

Our binger, on the other hand, who is constantly on a diet, will eat sparingly at her evening meal, preparing grilled fish with steamed broccoli and carrots and avoiding the mashed potato she serves to her partner and children. She too may serve apple pie for dessert, but only to the other members of the family. Unfortunately, one of her children may leave the crust of his pie and she absent-mindedly pops this into her mouth. This activates the need for more of the same and she will quickly finish the rest of the pie, then nibble on biscuits while clearing up. Later, preparing the children's lunch boxes for the following day, she will open a five-pack of chocolate biscuits, put one into each box and eat the remaining three. Now into full binge-mode, she will continue eating for the whole evening, often indulging in weird food combinations like spooning lemon curd and muesli into a tin of condensed milk and eating it out of the tin with a teaspoon (as you do). She will do this stealthily, keeping an eye on the door in case anyone should come in and see her. She *knows* why she is fat and tells herself she will 'start her diet again tomorrow'.

Changing Bad Eating Patterns

When you are greatly overweight, your 'fat' becomes the problem and your lack of control both mystifying and depressing. Some doctors classify this as an obsessive-compulsive phenomenon but the issue is the overeating, not the result. You need to identify the problem behaviourally rather than in terms of your appearance.

The best way to deal with this is to give up the notion of dieting (even 'sensible dieting' is a contradiction in terms) and substitute a healthy-eating plan encompassing food from every group and cutting out only the food that is not good for your health. Eating is something to be enjoyed rather than feared. A balanced diet is not a biscuit in each hand.

In a following chapter I will show you how to change the words that have made you fat in the past and substitute them for words that will keep you slim. As you are the one who talks to yourself, you are the only one who hears what you say, so you need to keep it positive all the time. This may sound easy, but if you have been a compulsive eater for many years, you are so used to berating yourself about your uncontrolled eating, your perceived weakness and unacceptable shape that these thoughts are a part of who you are. Subconsciously, you may want to hang on to them. Life is much simpler when all roads lead to one destination. You perceive that if all of your problems can be reduced to food and fat, the only solution is to go on a diet.

When you mentally shout at yourself for overeating, you get upset then need to comfort yourself with more food, thereby creating a circuit. If you stop being nasty to yourself and change your words to praise and encouragement, you break the circuit and stop translating all problems into fat. Faced with loads of problems, you'll need to come up with solutions instead, and sometimes that isn't easy. Let's face it: it is often fear of your real problems that sends you scurrying for the food in the first place.

Body-image Versus Self-image

It is time to stop confusing your body-image with your self-image. Body-image is not what you see in the mirror: it is the reaction you have within you in response to what you see. I understand that you want to be different from the way you are now – that you don't like the shape of your body – but this does not make you a bad person. You say you hate yourself but *you* are not your body. Consider your character: I am sure you are kind, generous, funny, a good loyal friend. What has that got to do with the fact that for some reason you have eaten too much food and allowed your body to become fat? Some of my very large clients say they feel ashamed to be seen and think that other people are talking about their size. So what? That is their problem. Why should you care? They don't live with you.

I am not suggesting you resign yourself to being overweight but that you acknowledge *what is* – without judging that reality. Acceptance does not imply self-delusion. When you accept yourself you simply say, 'This is how I am right now and it's OK'. How you look, the number on the scales and your eating habits are neither good nor bad. They just are. As you learn a healthier way of eating, your body will reflect this change and you will get slimmer. For now, however, developing an acceptance of how you look is crucial to resolving your problem with food.

✻   The easiest thing to be in the world is you.   ✻
The most difficult thing to be is what other people want you to be.

The logic of why you binge may still elude you but that logic is there nonetheless. Each person in the course of their development finds ways of coping with life's experiences. Therefore your eating has simply become your chosen way of dealing with your problems. When you reach for food to comfort yourself, you are reaching back in time. It is something you have always done. So? Is that a reason to hate yourself? Of course not. What you are going to do now is to replace this means of coping with something better, and make the decision that from now on you are going to be nice to yourself.

What We are Going to Do

The aim of this book is to help you identify the foods, thoughts and behaviours that are keeping you fat so that you can make the necessary changes. I want to make you feel better about yourself – not simply to lose weight no matter what it takes. This means that the plan you devise should not be geared towards undereating – or trying to achieve a negative energy balance. Rather, if you can eliminate overeating – meaning eating in excess of your body's natural requirements – and learn to stay in control, your problem will be solved.

Your objective, instead of focusing on the numbers on a scale, is to develop healthy and sustainable eating and exercise habits, and build a more positive body image. Here are some of the issues we will be addressing in the following chapters:

Step 1: What is Your Specific Goal?

Not a dream, but a real goal, a target you can reasonably achieve? Of course it's fine to dream ('I wish I could eat as much as I like and still be slim') but a goal is something you want to achieve and are prepared to work towards. Is it only your weight that you want to change or some other aspect of your life? What is really keeping you fat? What do you need to change? Be realistic in your answers.

If your goal is to be permanently slim, what are you prepared to sacrifice to achieve this? You now know that you can't eat everything you want any time you want it. Are you prepared to live without the sort of food you know is not good for your health and shape and just con-centrate on putting healthy food into your body?

Step 2: How Do You Intend to Measure Your Progress?

Are you aiming to stay below a certain weight or go for a dress size at which you feel comfortably slim? Again, make this something that is achievable, not wishful thinking.

Step 3: Devise an Eating Plan

This should be a plan you can live with, not too far removed from the way you eat now. I will help you do that in the next couple of chapters. Arrange your environment in such a way that it helps you achieve the results you want. This means making your house and your workplace 'safe'; stocking up your fridge and freezer with healthy food; and planning an exercise routine that you can stick with on a regular basis. Rely on your strategy, planning and programming, not on your willpower.

Step 4: Assess the Obstacles

To pursue a goal seriously requires you to assess the obstacles realistically and create a strategy for dealing with them. Identify those places, times, situations, other people and circumstances that set you up for failure. Reprogram those diversions so they cannot compete with what you really want. This means getting to know when you are likely to be tempted, and working out your own plan to deal with it. For example, if you always pop into the bakery for a Danish pastry on your way to work, find an alternative route. Avoid buying your evening newspaper in a shop where they also sell sweets and chocolates. If crisps set you off, tell your children not to eat them in front of you.

Step 5: Define Your Goal in Short, Measurable Steps

A wishful-thinking statement would be, 'I am aiming to go from a size 16 to a size 8 by the summer'. A reality-based statement would be, 'I will make the necessary changes to enable me to lose one pound a week for the next 20 weeks'. Changes happen one step at a time.

If you think about losing four dress sizes, the task can seem overwhelming. But it looks decidedly manageable when you break it down into the steps of losing one or two pounds a week. Steady progress through well-chosen, realistic stages produces lasting results in the end. But you have to know what those steps are before you set out.

Step 6: Be Accountable for Your Actions or Non-actions

As they progress towards their goal, people tend to con themselves and think, 'That little bit won't hurt' or 'It's raining, I'll go for my walk later'. Some people find it helpful to share their plan with a trusted friend to whom they have to report their progress periodically. The thought that someone is checking up on them might prevent a tempting situation from turning into a binge. If you think this will work for you, then go for it.

Personally, I usually advise people not to confide in others, mainly to avoid the sort of remarks people feel obliged to trot out whenever anyone is on a diet, such as 'Why? You don't need to lose weight' or 'Oh, come on, try a bit of this, it's not fattening'. It is nobody's business when you put on weight and nobody's business when you lose it.

Step 7: Lose the 'Diet' Mentality

If everyone stopped talking about eating, weight and body shape all the time, it might cease to be such an important and debilitating issue in our lives. We might also find many more interesting things to talk about. So how about:

★ Don't compliment friends when they look like they've lost weight.

★ Don't whinge about how much weight you have put on so your friends feel they have to say that you don't look as though you have.

★ When the conversation turns to weight and eating habits, start talking about something else – books, films, how there is nothing to watch on television.

★ Cut out all the negative, guilt-ridden comments about food ('I ate so much last night!'), including your habit of berating yourself for overeating ('I am such a pig').

That last point is extremely important. I understand that you want to be different from the way you are now. I also know that, ironically, accepting yourself as you are is a prerequisite for changing. This means accepting your body in its current shape and not putting yourself down all the time. Hating the way you look sends you scurrying to the fridge. Possibly your self-hatred is the factor most responsible for keeping you fat.

Get ready to programme yourself for success.

Conversation with Client

C: *How can I get rid of cellulite?*

Me: *You can't.*

C: *Is that it?*

Me: *Is that what?*

C: *The end of the conversation?*

Me: *What do you want me to say? Have you tried to get rid of cellulite?*

C: *Are you kidding?! I've tried everything. I've rubbed in creams, lotions, radioactive mud and seaweed extract. I've had pads strapped to my thighs with electric currents going through them. I've been wrapped in tight bandages and enveloped in hot wax. My bum has been squished between rollers and I've even had electrodes put in under the skin into the actual fat…*

Me: *Ouch! What does that do?*

C: *An electric current passes between each pair of positive/negative needles and it's meant to make the fat cells fight each other.*

Me: *And do what? Jump out and run away? Oh please! How did that work for you?*

C: *It didn't.*

Me: *Then get real. You cannot break down fat from the outside. It has to go through the process of lipolysis within your body to be turned into a form that can be used as energy. Look, you are eating sensibly, you're losing weight, your legs are getting toned from all the exercise, so just relax and enjoy life.*

C: But the cellulite is still there.

Me: Then learn to love it – because it sure loves you. Why else would it stay with you all this time? Because it's very attached to you, that's why!

C: Smartarse!

Conversation with Client

C: I have always believed in taking extra vitamins and minerals to ensure I get a balanced diet. Am I right?

Me: Most people who take vitamins do so as a protection against various ailments, but vitamin pills do not 'cure' anything. Neither does not taking them make you susceptible to illness. Vitamins are components of food and are found in plants and animals. If you are eating food from all the main food groups, you shouldn't need to take anything extra. On the other hand, some of the food we buy is so adulterated and processed that much of the vitamin content is lost.

C: Is that a No?

Me: That depends. What are you taking?

C: I take calcium for my bones, magnesium, vitamins E and C, gelatin for my brittle nails, vitamin B6 for premenstrual thingy, garlic pills, that stuff that improves your memory – what's it called? – um – anyway, I take iron *in case I'm anaemic, aloe vera, lecithin to break down my fat...*

Me: *Hang on a minute. You take lecithin to what?*

C: *Really! You're a diet counsellor – you should know this! I want to get thinner and I read that lecithin breaks down fat.*

Me: *Oh it does indeed, but only in the food that you eat as an aid to digestion, not the fat already encasing your thighs. Lecithin is an emulsifier. It breaks down the fat you eat into tiny droplets and carries them in the blood to the tissues that need it. It doesn't obligingly break it down and shunt it out of your body! Anyway, your body makes all the lecithin you need and if you take extra, your body will simply make less.*

C: *How disappointing. But surely everybody needs extra vitamin D because there is so little sunshine in this country, and I also take royal jelly because it's supposed to have magical properties.*

Me: *Rubbish! Royal jelly is made by bees to make queen bees strong. Royal jelly capsules are made by humans to make money. Why are you taking all this stuff? Wouldn't it be better simply to eat lots more healthy food?*

C: *(shrugging) Can't afford it.*

Chapter Three

The Sugar You Eat is the Fat You Wear

'Woe is she who partaketh most plentifully of the fruit of the sugar cane,' sayeth the prophet Tatenlyle (from the Book of Diabetes, Type 2, verse 1). 'For verily, this will bestow upon her the gift of mighty generous thighs that overflow her airline seat and render unto her much embarrassment.'

So – let me ask you: have you got a large hippocampus? If the answer is: 'Well, it was the last time I looked', you may be mistaken. Eating an abundance of sugary food can enlarge just about every part of your body but could be shrinking the part of your brain that deals with memory – the hippocampus.

According to research carried out by Dr Antonio Convit at the New York University School of Medicine, higher-than-normal blood sugar levels can cause the hippocampus to reduce in size. People with raised blood sugar were shown to perform less well in short-term memory tests than those with normal blood sugar levels.

Some of us do not have enough insulin – the hormone that removes sugar from the blood – to deal with all the sugary cakes and chocolate bars we put away. As a result, sugar collects in the blood instead of being pumped to body tissues such as the brain, where it is needed as fuel. As Dr Convit explained, when the hippocampus is looking for that extra fuel during memory processing and can't find what it needs, it ends up shrinking.

Now, what was I saying? Oh yes, moving down from the hippocampus to the parts where that sugar will ultimately settle…

My Story

Like many people, I used to grab for food whenever I felt anxious, stressed or bored. Starting with cake or biscuits, I would resign myself to the fact that I had 'broken my diet'. This meant that I might as well go on stuffing my face with food and restart my diet the next day. Then I would gravitate towards chocolate and ice cream. After a while, as the sweet taste became more cloying, I would switch to savoury foods, usually crisps or nuts, washed down with gallons of cold fizzy drinks like diet (!) cola.

Once fully into binge-mode, all thoughts of healthy food would disappear. While serving dinners of chicken or fish I had cooked for the rest of the family, I would make a pile of toast, layer on the butter and cheese and plough through the lot, before heading back to the cake and chocolate – dessert time!

The next day I would wake in a terrible state: horribly bloated, lethargic and deeply depressed. With my clothes feeling tight and uncomfortable to remind me of what I had done, I would try and analyse why I kept doing this while knowing throughout that it would make me feel so awful. I couldn't understand my own behaviour. I certainly had no wish to be fat. All I knew was that once the sugar craving took hold, I gave in to it every time.

A binge would usually last about three days before I could get myself back on my 'diet', whatever popular pro-gramme I was attempting to follow. As this was a long time ago, it was probably the Beverley Hills diet or the F-Plan.

My weight used to fluctuate by about a stone. I kept three sets of clothes, from skinny-mini skirts to saggy-baggy sweat pants, to cover all eventualities. Most aston-ishing, though, was the extent to which my eating habits affected my mood. When I was slim and eating normal meals I felt light, happy and confident. I would exercise regularly and was fit, supple and strong. After a binge, however, I felt heavy and depressed. Even hauling myself out of bed was a massive effort. I hated being fat and hated myself for being fat. I had no inclination to go near the gym and was sure that if I ran my thighs would jiggle like a mobile waterbed. I was either bad-tempered and snappy or just limp and weepy. The slightest problem upset me enormously and I had an overwhelming sense of being out of control and unable to cope – not only with my food choices but with everything.

Why should this be? If I struggled into some jeans and the two sides of the zip refused even to make eye contact, let alone meet and engage, I could see why that might be dispiriting, but surely not enough to produce the sort of depression that was affecting my whole life.

Enlightenment came when someone recommended a book called *Sugar Blues* published in 1975 by the American author, William Dufty. Reading it produced a 'lightbulb moment' for me. Dufty described how he was extremely overweight, had no energy and suffered recurring irritations like migraine, bloating and stomach problems, bleeding gums and haemorrhoids and often felt low with depression. He wrote: 'One night I read a book that said if you are sick, it is your own damn fault. You know better than anyone else how you have been abusing your body, so stop it.'

Sugar, said Dufty, is a poison, 'more lethal than opium and more dangerous than atomic fallout'. He resolved to stop eating it. He then went through his kitchen cupboards reading the food labels and was shocked to discover that once he threw out any products that contained refined sugar, the shelves were almost bare.

Starting his new eating regime, Dufty suffered withdrawal symptoms for 24 hours but then described a feeling of being 'reborn'. Over the next few weeks his depression lifted, he lost 200lb (imagine what he must have weighed before!), his skin improved and the various ailments he had suffered from gradually disappeared.

Could a food as innocuous and as readily available as sugar really cause a mental condition like depression? It seemed unlikely. I began studying the effects of sugar in more depth and was privileged to meet the late Professor John Yudkin, Professor of Nutrition and Dietetics at London University. He urged me to read his book *Pure, White and Deadly*, about the scourge of refined sugar. Reading it produced another 'lightbulb moment': I was convinced.

I made the decision to stop eating foods containing sugar. Initially, it was incredibly difficult. I found it practically impossible to bring up children in a sugar-free environment, and I had five of them, all great fans of chocolate biscuits. However, once I made that commitment to stop, I gradually lost the taste for sugar. I still can't believe I am actually writing that sentence 30 years later. It took about three weeks to get it out of my system but I stopped bingeing, the scales gradually went down a stone and stabilized at the lower weight and my niggling depression disappeared.

Once I became free of what I thought of as the 'black hole' inside me that was my sugar craving, I realized what a difference this made to my life. I am a completely different person when I am not eating sugar. On the odd occasion when, under extreme stress, I have eaten some sugary item, the depression comes straight back.

Obviously this won't be the same for everyone. The vast majority of people take sugar in some form every day and are not depressed as a result. When I use the word 'depression' in this instance I am not referring to the sort of clinical depression that necessitates the use of drugs to control it, but a persistent negative state of mind that pulls you down and makes the simplest task a gigantic effort.

Some enlightened people are catching on. Comedian Victoria Wood admitted that her bottom was once so big she needed planning permission before putting on her knickers. She said in an interview that she shed two stone simply by giving up all foods containing sugar and now wouldn't touch it again. The singer Geri Halliwell was even more strident in her views. 'Sugar is like cocaine for me,' she stated in a television interview, 'Once I start, I cannot stop eating it and it makes me feel dreadful.'

> You are allergic to sugar – it makes you break out in fat.

Sugar: the Facts

I'll tell you about sugar and you can decide for yourself.

Sugar is produced by harvesting and processing sugar cane, which grows in tall, bamboo-like plants, and sugar beet, which is a root crop. If you were to chew on raw sugar cane, you would be taking in some fibre, vitamins and minerals, but once the manufacturing process is complete and those bamboo shoots become white crystals, they contain zero nutrients. The same can be said of processing wholemeal flour into white flour and wholegrain rice into white rice; the fibre and vitamin content are lost.

Sugar manufacturers continue to promote sugar as a 'natural' substance on the basis that sweet foods have been eaten for centuries in the form of honey and berries. However, there is a world of difference between a bowl of sweet red strawberries and a chocolate bar. So how natural is natural? Has anyone seen a doughnut tree?

Sugar Marketing

More than £100 million is spent each year on marketing and advertising sweets and sugary foods, especially during children's television programmes, presenting these products as desirable and readily attainable to this key target audience. The Food Commission study, which examined 39 hours of viewing, found that nearly 40 per cent of commercials shown during children's programmes are for food products, most of them high in fat or sugar. Hence the rise of what the manufacturers and advertisers call 'pester power', where the children dictate what goes into the supermarket trolleys.

You can just imagine the brainstorming session at a chocolate manufacturer:

'OK guys, now how can we get people to eat more chocolate?'

'What about a promotion aimed at children? We could put a voucher in every bar and when they have collected a certain number, they'll get a prize.'

'Sounds good – what sort of prize?'

'I've got it! We'll offer sports equipment for schools! How about that? In that way we're also encouraging kids to do more sport. We can even get the Sports Minister to endorse it!'

'Brilliant idea!'

Pay rises and bonuses for the creative team.

And so it came about that in April 2003 the Sports Minister, Richard Caborn, gave his blessing to Cadbury's 'Get Active' campaign by saying, 'I am delighted Cadbury is prepared to support this drive to get more young people active by providing equipment and resources for schools. This could make a real difference to the quality of young people's lives.'

It could well do that! The Food Commission worked out that a child would have to eat 170 chocolate bars costing £71 to get a £10 basketball. These snacks would contain around 38,463 calories and just over 2kg of fat. To work that off would only take about 90 hours of basketball.

For the cricket fans, a set of cricket equipment would require vouchers from at least 2,730 chocolate bars containing more than 600,000 calories and including more than 33kg of fat — that's about the size and weight of a ten-year-old child. By the time the kiddies had chomped their way through that lot, they would be too fat to use the equipment anyway.

A few months later, after much criticism by health groups and teachers, Cadbury sheepishly announced that the vouchers would be valid until April 2004 when the scheme would be 'reviewed' – i.e. scrapped.

Childhood obesity is soaring. Surveys in early 2003 classified 31 per cent of children as overweight and 17 per cent obese, according to the British Dietetic Association. Health campaigners are extremely worried about the way the multinational confectionery companies with vast marketing budgets are bypassing parents and classrooms to aim directly at children through their computers and mobile phones. The internet is also being used as a front-line marketing tool, where online games are based around confectionery and children are encouraged to e-mail each other with the games in so-called 'viral marketing'.

None of these companies is doing anything illegal and the Food and Drink Federation is unabashed. As its deputy director-general says, 'Let's be clear about this: children are consumers. They have spending power. They are advertised to. It is perfectly legitimate.' Manufacturers also have no qualms about using celebrities to promote their products: Britney Spears promoted Pepsi, S Club 7 sold Cadbury's chocolate and Sooty helped to sell Milky Bar white chocolate. Even Harry Potter has been signed up by Mars and Coca-Cola.

School children are being bribed with burgers and fries to stop them playing truant. One universal fast-food company is running a project which offers schools free meal vouchers, which teachers use to reward children who turn up or try hard. Several schools have taken them up.

Junk Food Can Cause Health Problems

The rapid escalation of obesity in all developed countries is so worrying that in May 2003, Dr Gro Harlem Brundtland, director general of the World Health Organization (WHO), called a meeting of the six main companies involved in the food and drinks industry to discuss the threat posed by junk food. Dr Brundtland asked the companies to reduce the levels of sugar, salt and saturated fats in many of their products, as well as to work on educating their customers about dietary issues. The meeting was in response to WHO scientists who warned of an explosion in diet-related deaths and illnesses in the coming years unless consumers change their eating habits.

The scientists' report recommended that only 10 per cent of our calorie intake should come from sugar and 10 per cent from saturated fat. At present, many single food items, such as a ready-made meal or large chocolate bar, contain more than this recommended allowance. A survey of the eating habits of children aged between four and eighteen found that they were eating double this amount of sugar and saturated fat. More than 80 per cent of the children questioned in the survey, by the Office for National Statistics, said the food they ate most were crisps, biscuits, chocolate, white bread, chips, pizza and hamburgers.

Initially, the WHO's picture of sugar, fat and salt as a triumvirate of evils drew furious protests from the food industry who insisted that 25 per cent was a safe limit, and tried to rubbish the WHO's scientific analysis. But as a representative from the International Obesity Task Force said, 'I don't know any mother who would want a quarter of the food on her baby's plate to be sugar. It's ridiculous.'

The United States have emphatically rejected the WHO's recommendations to discourage the consumption of fatty, sugary food through education, pricing and restrictions on advertising. William Steiger, a US Health Department official, told the WHO's executive board in Geneva that Washington wanted less emphasis on regulation and more on individual responsibility. He insisted there was no firm evidence that sugary and high-calorie processed food was the main cause of obesity. Really? This couldn't be because the food and sugar industries are significant donors to the Republican Party, could it? No, no, of course not. Anyway, why would Americans need advice on healthy eating? They are the slimmest, healthiest people in the world, aren't they?

However, several British firms, to their credit, pledged to reduce or eliminate the use of hydrogenated vegetable fat and oil from their products. Also known as trans fatty acids, hydrogenated vegetable fats and oils are linked to the build-up of LDL cholesterol, which is associated with obesity, clogging of the arteries, heart disease and strokes. Cadbury, Kellogg, Nestlé and United Biscuits, makers of McVitie's biscuits, all agreed to change the recipes of their biscuits, chocolate snacks and cereals to make them more healthy.

Well, I guess that's a start but all the manufacturers are keeping very quiet about the amount of sugar in their products, probably hoping that by giving in on the fat issue this will divert people's attention away from the sugar. The manufacturers can say quite legitimately that a moderate intake of sweet food is not harmful but, for reasons that I will show you, the way many of us respond physiologically to processed sugar products means that moderation is simply not possible. Do you know anyone who can eat just one chocolate peanut?

Sugar Addiction

◌ **If there is a food you can't control, then that** ◌
food is controlling you.

Research has verified that sugar can be addictive. John Hoebel, a professor of psychology at Princeton University in New Jersey, showed that rats fed a diet containing 25 per cent sugar were thrown into a state of anxiety when the sugar was removed. Their symptoms, including chattering teeth and shaking, were similar to those seen in humans suffering withdrawal from nicotine or morphine.

Dr Hoebel writes that foods high in fat and sugar trigger the brain to release natural substances called opioids that stimulate the production of the 'pleasure chemical' dopamine. The implication is that some animals – and by extension some people – can become overly dependent on sweet food, thereby causing the brain to become addicted to its own opioids. Drugs give a stronger effect, but it is essentially the same process. When the rats were given a synthetic blocker to stop sugar-stimulated opioids, their dopamine levels fell in the same way that they would when, for example, heroin is withdrawn.

More research on sugar addiction has been carried out at the University of Wisconsin Medical School, where the neuroscientist Ann Kelley has revealed that the release of such sugar-induced opioids seems to encourage people to eat more sugary foods, even when they are not hungry. Again, the study focused on rats but Kelley says that the changes in their brain chemistry are equivalent to that of humans. The rats were given a small taste of sweet food then two bowls were set down, one containing healthy food and the other containing more of the sweet stuff. Guess which bowl the rats chose?

You have to decide what is important – eating sugary food or being slim. You can't do both.

What Sugar Does to Your Body

When you eat foods containing refined sugar, such as cakes, biscuits, chocolate, sweets and desserts, the sugar level – or rather the glucose level – in your blood rises rapidly. To deal with this your pancreas produces a hormone called insulin to clear the sugar out of the bloodstream and direct it into the body cells. Some of the sugar is directed to your muscles to be used for immediate energy; some of it goes to the liver to be stored in the form of glycogen for future energy; and the rest gets **stored in your fat cells**. Hellooo?

Your digestive system was not designed to deal with large amounts of sugary foods, especially on an empty stomach, so when you overeat in this way, your pancreas is stimulated to produce too much insulin. This causes your blood sugar level to drop sharply. A little while after eating your chocolate bar, you will still have some insulin circulating in your bloodstream, searching for something to work on and causing a craving for – yes, you've guessed it – more sugar.

What you eat right now will affect what you eat for the rest of the day.

Therefore insulin is the hunger hormone. If you eat a lot of sugary food, you are *programming yourself to be hungry most of the time*. You are also programming your body to become a fat-storing machine. Insulin not only stores fat, a risk factor for Type 1 diabetes, it also appears to damage artery walls, making it easier for cholesterol and fat to stick, build up and cause heart disease.

Be under no illusions: sugar is your enemy. It makes you fat, tired, bloated, lethargic, depressed (in some cases) and can rot your teeth. It contains no vitamins or minerals and has no nutritional value. If a new food were advertised with these attractive features, would you buy it?

Hypoglycaemia

I used to feel a bit dizzy sometimes after eating a high-sugar snack, especially on an empty stomach. A glucose-tolerance test showed that I was suffering from mild hypoglycaemia (low blood sugar). It was scary but not serious. This condition is caused by the body trying to rebalance itself after a surge of insulin, producing glucose from the glycogen stores in the liver to mop up the excess insulin. When this happens, adrenaline is also produced, and this tends to exacerbate the symptoms, causing lethargy and weakness. These are further worsened if you eat at irregular intervals, leave long gaps between meals and then grab a sugary snack instead of a balanced meal. Apparently, drinking lots of tea and coffee can also stimulate the release of insulin, as can smoking.

Further studies, reported in *New Scientist* magazine, show that while appetite is thought to be controlled by a complex system of hormones and other substances produced by the body, large doses of sugar (delivered by a single fast-food meal) can over-ride this system. It appears to take only one such meal to raise the production of galanin, a protein made in the brain that influences eating by increasing the body's preference for fats and sugary carbohydrates.

Most people think you 'need' a certain amount of sugar to give you energy. However, the chief source of energy for your muscles, kidneys, brain and nervous system is glucose, produced when your liver processes fats and carbohydrates into a form that your body can use. These need not include refined sugar.

The Glycaemic Index

Sugar is also central to the concept of the Glycaemic Index, something I have been struggling to understand for some time. The Glycaemic Index, referred to as GI, is the measure of which foods cause the blood sugar level to shoot up rapidly (bad), and which foods are digested and absorbed slowly, giving the pancreas time to dribble out the required amount of insulin to deal with it without the high/low surge (good).

So far, so good. Obviously, the least healthy food is pure sugar, which will cause the highest and fastest rise in blood glucose levels. Other foods are assessed as a percentage of the increase caused by pure sugar, creating this sliding scale or index. Rapidly digested foods have a high GI, whereas slowly digested food, which is more desirable for weight loss and health, has a low GI. Fruit, containing the natural sugar fructose, causes only 10 per cent of the rise of refined white sugar, thereby ensuring its place in the low GI category.

Apparently, the more high-GI foods you eat, the greater your total glucose 'load'. This is the sum of all the glucose released from foods that either contain sugar or convert to sugar in the body. The higher your load, the more you will experience high/low swings in blood sugar levels and cravings. *But* – and this is where my struggle comes in – wholemeal bread, brown rice and Shredded Wheat, which I would have considered healthy foods, are classified as high GI, whereas ice-cream made with cream and sugar is listed in the low GI column! Go figure, as they say…

Balancing Your Blood Sugar

Let's stick with proven facts: a mainly carbohydrate meal such as a baked potato, a sandwich made with white bread, pasta or risotto made with white rice will cause the same rapid rise in blood sugar as cakes and biscuits: 70–90 per cent. If you have protein with it, such as chicken in your sandwich, the effect will slow down a little and you will feel more full for longer. However, the faster the level goes up, the faster it will come down, leaving you hungry, tired and craving something sweet a little while later. That is why I advise you to restrict your intake of starchy carbohydrates during the day (not to zero: we are not Atkins fans here), and I will cover this topic more fully in the next chapter.

If you are looking for snacks that are low in sugar, be wary of so-called 'healthy' or 'natural' cereal bars. Check the labels carefully. The word 'organic' refers to the way the ingredients are grown or produced – it does not mean that the product is necessarily any less fattening than an ordinary chocolate bar or that it will contain any more fibre or fewer calories.

Some manufacturers try to avoid stating how much sugar is contained in their products by using a range of different names for sugar, such as corn syrup, dextrose or maltose. Honey is just as fattening and has the same high/low effect as sugar. Did you know that there are *nine* teaspoons of sugar in a Mars Bar? Would you deliberately create a snack for yourself using that amount of sugar?

Naturopaths suggest that we should emulate the diets of animals in the wild, like bears or monkeys who get their sweet taste from natural sources like berries and honey. That's all very well but monkeys and bears don't suffer from premenstrual tension as far as I know – or have a mother who says things like, 'I knew you were coming so I made your favourite chocolate brownies'.

Banish Tooth Decay

When I was a child there was a continuous supply of sweets and chocolates in the house. My mother was obviously a chocoholic and gave me sweets as a comfort when I was upset, as a treat to ensure I behaved, and whenever *she* ate them. Consequently my teeth were rotten from childhood until well into my 30s, full of fillings and crowns. When I decided to stop eating sugar because it was making me feel so awful, the miracle happened: I stopped getting tooth decay, which was certainly an unexpected bonus. Now when I go to the dentist, he cleans my teeth and I go home.

Just as people don't connect the food they eat with the shape it causes – that is, they will eat chocolate and crisps, drink plenty of alcohol and then wonder why they are fat – so we often don't connect eating sugar with tooth decay. Intellectually, you know that sugar rots your teeth because you have read it over and over again in magazines and newspapers. If you're spending an inordinate amount of time in the dentist's chair having fillings, root canal treatment, crowns and the occasional extraction, it is time to look at the contents of your sweetie cupboard – and your car…

Chocolate – the Ultimate Comfort Food

Surveys into women's eating habits reveal that chocolate is consistently the most craved sweet food. It was recently voted the UK's number 1 comfort food. Roasted cocoa contains 50 chemicals that can stimulate changes in body chemistry. Strangely, most of these are also found in large amounts in other high-fat foods like cheese and salmon, but these don't seem to be binge triggers. This is where emotion and texture play a part, as cheese and salmon hardly offer the same velvety sensation as a bar of chocolate. Chocolate also contains a substance called N-acylethanolamine, which produces a relaxing narcotic effect, and a chemical called phenylethylamine, which works the same way as an amphetamine to lift your mood and make you feel happy.

The amount of phenylethylamine in chocolate is much lower than in cheese and salmon, so why don't you crave a salmon sandwich? The answer is that we don't associate salmon with the same feelings. Women love chocolate because of its sensory properties. It tastes, smells and feels a particular way in the mouth, and women seem to have a very positive psychological association with this food. It can also lead to fierce discussions regarding the best brand, dark or milk, and whether it should be eaten soft and melty or cold and hard from the fridge. I can put an end to all debate here and now by declaring that Cadbury's milk chocolate is the best in the world and should be eaten at room temperature. But why doesn't it taste the same when bought abroad?

The only problem with eating a lot of chocolate, as we all know only too well, is that it can cause weight gain, depression and low self-esteem. For many of us, chocolate is 'the' sweet taste of choice. If you love the taste of chocolate and the good feeling it produces, this feeling gets imbued in your subconscious mind as a learned response. Possibly, like me, you were given sweets when young as a bribe or a reward for doing something good. Sweetness therefore becomes associated with pleasure, and when you don't feel good, you seek out something sweet to remedy it – thus developing the automatic craving for chocolate.

✌ **Get real! You like chocolate but it doesn't like** ✌
you.

The Beer Gut

Men don't escape the effects of eating massive amounts of junk food. This plays a part in forming the well-known beer belly. ('T-shirt shrunk in the wash' – yeah, right!) The gut contains friendly and unfriendly bacteria, and it's important to eat foods that keep the balance tipped in favour of the friendly type. These break down fat and help indigestible foods pass through the body. Good bacteria in the gut are killed off by too much sugar, while bad bacteria thrive on it – they just keep growing. Bad bacteria produce huge amounts of gas, which contributes to the bloated feeling of a big belly.

There are significant health risks from over-consumption of sugar. Sugar blunts your taste and is simply a form of empty calories that turns to fat. If you stuff yourself with sweets or junk food and drink a lot of alcohol you are unlikely to have any appetite for healthy food like fish, chicken or vegetables. If you keep eating like that, you are in danger of depriving your body of the nutrients and fibre that keeps it healthy.

Syndrome X

Given my own severe reaction to sugar, I make sure I keep up to date with any medical reports that add to my research. In March 2003, a group of doctors from all over the world held a conference in Monte Carlo to discuss a prevalent disorder affecting fatter people: insulin-resistance syndrome, also known as the metabolic syndrome and, more recently, Syndrome X. Insulin resistance is a condition in which the tissues of the body become progressively insensitive to the action of insulin, to the extent that more and more insulin is required to achieve normal blood glucose levels. This leads to higher levels of insulin circulating in the blood, obesity, high blood pressure, abnormal fat levels in the blood and Type 2 (adult-onset) diabetes. Sounds like fun.

Another complication of this syndrome is that excess fat and sugar, now converted into fat, are stored around the midriff, in the muscles, liver and pancreas. These fat deposits increase insulin resistance, which in turn makes it more difficult for the body to process sugar and fat. Hence ever-higher concentrations of insulin are needed to achieve the same biological effect.

Syndrome X is now acknowledged as an epidemic in the United States. According to Greg Critser, author of *Fat Land*, American people are 'the fattest people on the face of the earth'. Critser himself is a glutton for statistics, but nevertheless some of those he throws up are quite staggering: 20 per cent of Americans are obese and five million − *five million* − are classified as 'morbidly obese', meaning they qualify for gastroplasty, or stomach-stapling.

When Size Does Matter

This is hardly surprising as anyone visiting America is amazed by the size of the food portions served as standard in most restaurants. A regular serving of McDonald's fries has increased from 200 calories in 1960 to 610 in 2003. Likewise, American teenagers think nothing of ordering a 64-ounce cola drink known as the Big Gulp. That is more than three pints! Apparently, it is now perfectly conventional for Pizza Hut or Coca-Cola to pay individual high schools $100,000 a year for exclusive rights to sell their products on campus.

Understandably, diabetes is now the fastest-growing disease in America, with sales of insulin increasing by 24 per cent a year. 'These days, you've got to be in diabetes', a public relations executive for the Lilly drug company tells Critser.

However incredible the statistics from America, we should not get too complacent. Jumbo-size portions of hamburgers, cookies and muffins are becoming as common in the UK as the United States – the so-called 'portion distortion'. Doctors blame growing meal sizes on the 'value marketing' principle, whereby supermarkets, restaurants and cinemas encourage people to buy huge packets of crisps, king-size chocolate bars and triple-pack sandwiches. One 'meal deal', a popular lunch option for office workers, comprising a triple layer sandwich, crisps and a drink, can contain more than half the recommended daily calorie intake.

The extra food content costs the manufacturer very little but, to the consumer, it represents 'good value' and is highly enticing. When people are served more food, they eat more food, as shown in America where people are 'super-sizing' meals in their homes as well.

Studies have shown many diners fail to notice when they are given larger portions. In a recent experiment, when diners were given four differently sized portions of macaroni cheese on different days, fewer than half noticed the change. Those who took part in the study unwittingly consumed 30 per cent more calories on the days when they were served the largest portion.

The food industry has defended its record, claiming larger portions give consumers 'more choice'. Martin Paterson, of the Food and Drink Federation, said, 'Larger packs are not always consumed by one person or at one session, and parents can now often choose mini-products and multipacks.'

However, larger portions, often eaten while watching television, produce an automatic hand-to-mouth motion, which continues until the food is gone. Two children, sharing a 1.5-litre bottle of cola – either of the popular brands – will be ingesting 42 teaspoons of sugar between them.

It doesn't seem to occur to American people that the amount they eat is the cause of their obesity; they have no idea what constitutes a normal portion of food. There has to be another reason. This is why American scientists are very excited at having isolated an 'obesity gene'. Apparently, if you have inherited this fat gene, you could be susceptible to becoming overweight. Hey, isn't that great?! It's not your fault then, Lard-Butt, it's your genes!

Only – isn't it amazing how this particular gene has suddenly materialized in the last decade or so? Obviously

American evolution is different from, say, Ethiopian evolution because nobody seems to have the fat gene there.

Health Implications of Syndrome X

Yes, the Americans are paying the price for these supersized meals with obesity and chronic disease. Sadly, a similar price will be paid by Britons if action is not taken soon. Researchers at Leeds Metropolitan University say that Syndrome X is already affecting one in five British people. This is diagnosed when a patient has at least three of a group of biochemical problems including obesity, a low level of the good high-density cholesterol, blood pressure over 130/85 and the results of a fasting plasma glucose test over 6mmol/l. Alternatively, you could simply measure around your waist with a tape measure! Women's waists should measure below 32 inches (81cm) and they are at risk once they exceed 35 inches (89cm). Men's waist measurements should be below 37 inches (94cm) and they are at risk once they exceed 40 inches (101cm).

Syndrome X is caused by a diet high in saturated fats and refined sugars and carbohydrates. This changes the body chemistry so that it becomes insulin-resistant and cannot process sugar and fat efficiently. Alarmingly, according to a study at Derriford hospital in Plymouth, this condition is affecting some overweight children as young as five, who are showing early signs of developing Type-2 diabetes, normally only found in middle-aged people. Professor Terry Wilkins, who is leading the study, said, 'High insulin resistance is a ticking time bomb that almost always leads to diabetes. In 30 per cent of the children we are monitoring, the fuse is well and truly lit. Some of these kids have probably been on a high-fat/high-sugar diet since they started on solids.'

The unavoidable conclusion is that eating a lot of sugary food will not only make you fat, but can also prevent your body from working properly. Combined with a lack of exercise, it can leave you vulnerable to any of the severe medical conditions mentioned earlier.

Is there any good news? Well, yes. The principle works the same in reverse. The doctors at the Monte Carlo conference concluded that the best way to counter the increase in Syndrome X was to encourage their patients to drastically reduce the amount of sugar they eat, to lose weight and take more exercise. Oh – really? No surprises there then.

Break Free from the Sugar Trap

Let's get personal: are you caught in the sugar trap? Are there certain high-fat, high-sugar foods you can't resist? Foods you try and avoid because you know they will make you fat or start you off on a binge? Check out the following:

★ Do you feel a meal is incomplete unless it ends with 'something sweet'?

★ Do you insist that you can't have a cup of tea without a biscuit?

★ When you see a particular food, do you crave it?

★ Do you ever say 'I'll just have one' or 'I'll just have a little bit' and yet are always unable to stick to that?

★ Have you ever eaten this food instead of a meal?

★ Do you ever eat this food even though you are not hungry?

★ Is this the food you have tried to give up when you went on a diet in the past?

★ Is this the food you are definitely eating when the weight goes back on?

How many times did you answer 'Yes'? Only you will know if you are caught in the sugar trap, and only you know if you need to break free for the sake of your health, your shape and your self-esteem. Any food you cannot control is controlling you.

So it's up to you. Hopefully, you have not reached a stage of obesity where you will be affected by Syndrome X. But if you make a conscious decision to stop eating any food containing refined sugar, you will discover that there are significant and immediate benefits, not least that your skin will look better, your eyes will be clearer and you will look slimmer and less bloated.

You will also find that food tastes better and you will have the energy to get out and be more active. It usually takes three weeks – 21 consecutive days – to get the sugar residue out of your system so that you lose the craving for it. After that, you will feel a surge of energy, a lifting of your spirits and you will be amazed at the difference in your appearance. You will also lose weight.

 ⚘ **Is that doughnut more important than your** ⚘
    health, shape or self-esteem? Of course not.

Sugar Substitutes

Note that I am talking about refined sugar. That doesn't mean you have to give up a sweet taste altogether. You can still use artificial sweeteners like aspartame, marketed as Canderel in the UK, and as Equal in America. If you don't like the idea of chemical sweeteners, use fructose, the natural sugar found in fruit. You will find this in packets in the supermarket next to the sugar, labelled 'fructose' or 'fruit sugar'. Fructose is *not* less calorific than ordinary sugar but because it is metabolized straight into the bloodstream without going through the liver, it will prevent the surge of insulin that you would get from ordinary sugar, so you won't get that addictive craving for more.

If you can't live without an occasional biscuit or sweet, try diabetic foods. In the UK, Boots do a great-tasting range. I bet you won't be able to taste any difference in their toffees. Again, be warned that diabetic food is *not* any less fattening than ordinary food. However, you won't be able to eat a lot of it because the sweetener used in place of sugar is usually sorbitol, which will cause violent diarrhoea if you eat too much. Like fructose, though, sorbitol does not encourage the surge of insulin that marks the addictive quality in sugar, so the occasional diabetic toffee should satisfy your craving for a sweet without triggering the need to polish off the rest of the packet.

Making the Decision to Change

If you really want to change your body from fat-storing to fat-burning, then cutting out sugar and limiting your intake of starchy carbohydrates is the best way to do it. Maintaining low insulin levels is the most important goal for keeping your weight down.

Only you can make this decision. It has to be a pre-meditated choice – just like giving up smoking. Sugar may not be as damaging as nicotine but, in its own way, can have a dramatic effect on your looks, your energy levels, your shape and the way you feel about yourself. You have to decide what is important. If you would consider yourself deprived without a chocolate fix every day, then make up your mind that you will just carry on as you are and accept being lumpy. That's fine. It would be very boring if everyone looked the same. It all depends on how much your appearance matters to you. Personally, I would rather be slim than eat chocolate. You have the same choice.

☾ **You cannot eat everything you want, any time ☾ you want and still be slim.**

Myth: If you don't allow yourself to have certain foods

that you love, you will feel deprived and these are the foods you will binge on.

Wrong. You will find it much easier not to have any of these foods than to try and limit them. Just having a small bite of something and getting the taste when you know there is lots more to be had – well, that is hard. Someone giving up alcohol is never advised to have a small shot of whisky at tea time.

Maybe you are a regular overeater or a serious binger. Either way, it has nothing to do with avoidance and everything to do with availability. The fattening foods you keep to hand are the ones you will focus on, seek out, head for when you feel tired, irritable, niggly or bored. That is why you have a weight problem – because you overeat the same foods every time. You are not depriving yourself by not eating sugar. It is *by* eating sugar that you are depriving yourself – of being the slim, attractive person you want to be.

You can only feel deprived if you think you are making a sacrifice. But what sort of a sacrifice is giving up a substance that makes you fat and miserable? Giving up sugar is a freedom, not a deprivation. No more dithering about what you should eat. You can eat everything – *unless* it contains sugar. How simple is that?

30 Days to Make a Difference

If you really want to make a difference in your life, set aside 30 days, starting on the first day of the month, to cut out all sugar from your diet. Don't dwell on the negative aspects (no need for any 'I'll miss you my lovely icy-creamy Ben & Jerry' nonsense). Just think of all the different, delicious foods out there waiting for you to try and enjoy. Try different vegetables – no, there isn't any sticky-toffee cauliflower. Go to your local supermarket and check out the ever-expanding range of low-calorie foods. Increase your repertoire of tastes. Read the labels, though, because these products are not all sugar-free.

As with giving up any addictive substance, you may experience sudden bouts of tiredness in the first few days because you are not giving your body the false bursts of energy it has grown to expect from your usual chocolate snacks. You may also experience cravings for something sweet at certain times if this is what you are used to. A couple of dates or a handful of sultanas should provide the necessary sweet taste. After three or four weeks, you will lose the taste for sugar and these cravings will disappear. I know you don't believe me at the moment but the only way to see if I am telling the truth is to try it.

The truth is, you don't like sugary food as much as you think you do. When you are bingeing on cakes, biscuits and chocolate, haven't you sometimes felt despair instead of enjoyment because you know what you are doing will make you fat? I know you may also feel a bit panicky at the thought of never eating chocolate again – but that is not what I am saying. I am *suggesting* that you *choose* not to eat chocolate *today* – that's all. You never actually lose the taste for sweet food – you know you would enjoy it if you ate it – but you reach a point where you are not bothered whether you have it or not. You really do lose the craving.

If you are still doubtful about giving up sugar, here is another benefit you might consider: many of my clients have reported that, along with sudden bursts of energy and a feeling of lightness, comes a new sense of happiness. As one client put it, 'It's as though a veil has been lifted. I never realized how much sugar was pulling me down!' That might sound strange but it's an experience borne out by clients – and myself – over the years. They report feeling as though they have shed some unwanted burden: their faces look fresher, their skin clearer, and there is no puffiness round their eyes. They have loads of energy and no cravings. Obviously this is very subjective and you have to complete the no-sugar month to discover the benefits for yourself.

Once you set your mind to it, you will be amazed how easy it becomes to bypass the temptations waiting by the checkout. You really do seem to lose the taste for sweet foods to the point where, if you were offered a bar of chocolate or a fresh, juicy peach, you would opt for the fruit. If you are one of the 'I can't believe that!' sceptics, then all I can say is, give it a go.

After one month, see how you feel. If you want to go back to your old ways, that's up to you. Just give it a try.

The lady at the next table in the café broke a sugar lump in half. 'See,' she said triumphantly to her companion, 'I only take half a lump of sugar in my tea now.' And she popped one half into her tea – and the other half into her mouth! (Is it me?)

Case Study

Gemma Norton, aged 39, mother of Archie 9, Ellie 7 and Bertie 3.

'Being a working mum, I sometimes cursed women's lib for ensuring that all women have earned the right to be permanently tired. I know I felt drained and exhausted most of the time and was always getting colds and irritating ailments like thrush.

'My sister finally dragged me to see a dietician who noted my symptoms and told me I was suffering from hypoglycaemia – low blood sugar. He said that if I didn't cut down on my sugar intake, I would be a prime candidate for diabetes. He read out a list of symptoms including insomnia, irritability, aggression, acute tiredness and exhaustion, impatience, anxiety, indigestion and excessive sweating when stressed. I was shocked to realize I had experienced most of those and assumed it was normal.

'He explained how sugars and simple carbohydrates screwed up my blood sugar and insulin levels, and that I was compensating by running largely on adrenaline, which wasn't doing my immune system much good. That was why I picked up every passing virus.

'I was determined to change my way of eating and cut out all foods containing refined sugar, as well as bread, pasta and potatoes. The first week was an absolute nightmare. I was permanently hungry, I thought about food all the time and my brain seemed to have packed up completely, even though I could eat any other food I wanted. I desperately craved my usual chocolate croissant with my morning cappuccino and my Kit Kat at tea time. I was so grumpy that no-one at the office dared speak to me. I really was an addict going through withdrawal, and the drug was sugar. It was only now, when I couldn't have it, that I realized I had unconsciously been topping up my energy levels with something sweet every two or three hours throughout the day.

'The most difficult time was eating with the children and stopping myself picking at their leftover food. Also, standing at the checkout in the supermarket eyeing the chocolates for what seemed like hours till it was my turn to pay.

'There was a marked breakthrough after day 10 when I suddenly began to feel much better. I slept soundly and woke up refreshed instead of needing two cups of coffee and a bagel to jog my brain into gear. My skin looked very clear and the puffiness round my eyes, which I thought was just part of me, disappeared. I felt much calmer during the day, less irritable and stressed, and still felt alert in the evenings instead of my eyes closing halfway through a TV programme.

'I have now done three weeks without sugar (and without thrush!), and my new way of eating has become the norm. I know what I am going to eat, I love my afternoon strawberries and sugar-free yoghurt and, amazingly, do not crave chocolate at all. The difference this has made to my life is incredible, and although I might glance at the desserts in the supermarket, I will not go back to eating them. It is too high a price to pay.'

Conversation with New Client, Sara, who Weighs 14 stone 11 pounds

Me: *So you agree that if you want to be slim there is no point in eating food that makes you fat?*

S: *Yes.*

Me: *You said you have always been a binger. Which is the first food you gravitate towards when your mind switches into binge-mode?*

S: *Cheesecake, pizza, chips, cream cakes, alcohol, ice cream, chunks of Yorkshire pudding dipped in sweet 'n' sour sauce, custard…*

Me: *No, just give me one thing that triggers a binge.*

S: *Harrods food hall.*

Me: *I don't think I am making myself clear here. Which food would you be prepared to give up in order to get slim?*

S: *Marmite.*

Me: *But Marmite isn't fattening.*

S: *I know. I hate it.*

Me: *Would you be prepared to stop eating sugar?*

S: *I never take sugar in tea – or coffee.*

Me: *I mean, all food containing sugar.*

S: *I don't know. All I know is I've got great fat arms and I desperately need to lose the flab round my middle. God, my hips are spreading so much they'll soon need their own postcode!*

Me: *Now answer the question.*

S: *I've forgotten what you asked.*

Me: *Are you always this indecisive?*

S: *Well, yes and no…*

Me: *I asked if you were prepared to stop eating foods containing sugar.*

S: *I suppose I could give it a try.*

Me: *'Giving it a try' isn't a commitment. If you are really serious about losing weight, you have to change your thinking about food and take on board the advice I give you.*

S: *I'll do it – if you guarantee it will get rid of the podgy bit just above my bra at the back. Look – even my knees are fat!*

Me: *You seem to be obsessed with the shape of your body.*

S: *Not at all. Do these earrings make my face look fat?*

Chapter Four

Your 'Living Slim' Eating Plan

Behold the words of the prophet Bulgythias (from the Book of Cellulite, Size 22, Bust 48C): 'And it shall come to pass, if thou dost deprive thine body of sustenance for two whole days, on the third day thou shalt surely binge.'

I hope we're agreed: changing the way you live now requires planning and strategy. The old haphazard 'going on a diet' without a concrete plan has failed every time. This time the emphasis is going to be on long-term slimness as opposed to a quick-fix weight loss.

Therefore, unlike every other weight-loss scheme, this plan does not advocate a 'diet' phase followed by a 'maintenance' phase – the latter, in most cases, meaning 'going back to the pattern of eating that made you fat in the first place'!

Choosing the Right Foods

Food is meant to enhance your life, not diminish it. You can't expect your brain to perform adequately if you don't feed it the right ingredients. The food you put in your stomach supplies the brain with the raw materials it needs to manufacture various hormones that affect your mood. Food can also directly influence the production of certain neurotransmitters – chemicals that pass messages through your nervous system – that lift your spirits and keep you feeling reasonably cheerful. Making the right food choices will prevent the dramatic highs and lows in blood sugar levels that lead to cravings and withdrawal symptoms.

Your choices, though, must be foods you enjoy so that both your body and mind recognize the experience of eating. The production of saliva and other digestive juices increases when you choose food you love, and this enhances your pleasure. When you go on a diet you may force yourself to eat food you don't particularly like because it is 'good for you' and then find that your sensory recognition mechanism switches off and you won't really feel like you've eaten. In addition, you have receptors in your jaw which respond when you chew, which is why diet foods such as replacement meal drinks don't really satisfy you.

There are also receptors in the stomach that send signals of fullness to the brain when food is present. Protein and high-fibre foods like wholegrain bread, vegetables and fruit have thick cell walls, which swell in the presence of water and send lots of messages to the brain, making you feel satiated. Sadly, sweet foods pass through the stomach without these receptors being activated.

This fact was borne out by experiments carried out by Dr Susan Jebb, of the Medical Research Council, working with volunteers from the United Kingdom and Africa. She showed that the amount of calories different foods contain weight for weight is a critical factor in regulating food intake. If calories are densely packed into a food, people may easily overdo their intake without realizing it. Dipping into a box of fudge, which is rich in sugar and fat, could cause your calorie intake to soar almost unnoticed. Conversely, when the food is not dense in calories and energy, as with a serving of broccoli, it is not going to be stuffed down uncontrollably. Dr Jebb found that energy density in the average British meal is two-and-a-half times higher than in a traditional African meal. The answer is to choose your food wisely at every meal. You don't need anyone to tell you which foods are fattening.

There is no such thing as low-fat crisps.

A Flexible Eating Plan

If you are used to eating a certain way, it's unlikely you would stick to a food plan that deviates drastically from what you know and like. Let's face it: you find it satisfying and comforting to eat for long periods of time. This is born out by your habit of nibbling on food for an entire evening. Therefore it makes sense to find a low-calorie source of food that will take a long time to eat without making you fat. A slice of cake containing 300 calories slips down in two minutes. The same number of calories in a huge salad would take half an hour and would satisfy all your tastes from crunchy carrots to sweet cherry tomatoes.

I have found, from many years of advising my over-weight clients, that the following method of eating seems to work for most people. It can be adapted to fit in with your existing way of eating as the choice of ingredients is entirely up to you.

This eating plan is meant to make you feel good – not to make you feel as though you are being punished for being too fat. You need to *eat*. You have been trying *not* to eat for long enough!

The rules are quite simple:

1. Decide not to eat any food containing refined sugar. You know what these foods are. No, you will not feel 'deprived' because this leaves you free to eat *everything else*.

2. Have protein at every main meal. Protein foods are milk, yoghurt, eggs, cheese, tofu, fish (including tuna, sardines, smoked salmon, tinned salmon, plaice, cod, halibut, shellfish etc.), chicken, duck, turkey, and meat such as lamb, beef and pork. Try and avoid processed meat like sausages, salt beef and salami, as these are packed with unhealthy preservatives.

3. Only have starchy carbohydrates at breakfast time and, if hungry, as an evening snack, not during the

day. The starchy carbs I am referring to are bread, potatoes, rice, pasta and pastry. If you are absolutely starving during the day or there is nothing else available, then rice cakes are OK – but only as an emergency food.

4. Fill up on fruit and vegetables. Vegetables, other than potatoes, can be eaten freely, raw or cooked at any time during the day as an accompaniment to protein or by themselves.

5. Have regular small meals throughout the day. Do not let three hours go by without eating something, even if it's only an apple. (Just do it, OK!)

6. Drink a large glass of water – eight big swallows – as soon as you wake up in the morning (keep a bottle by your bed) and several times during the day.

7. Alcohol is fattening. Try not to have more than one glass with your evening meal.

Let's go through these one by one and I'll explain the rationale behind this eating plan.

> Don't say 'I can't eat that because I'm on a diet'. Say 'I choose not to eat that because I know it's bad for me'.

Rule 1: Cutting out Sugar

You do not need me to list the foods that contain refined sugar! The obvious ones are cakes, biscuits, sweets, chocolate, ice cream and desserts. If you are unsure, read the labels: maltose, dextrose, corn syrup, glucose, sucrose, lactose, honey – sorry, those are all sugar, even when disguised as 'organic sweeteners' (do the manufacturers really think we are that stupid?!). Fructose is the only acceptable sugar if it is the sole sweetening agent listed, but this is rarely the case!

The order of ingredients is also important. The nearer each ingredient is to the top of the list, the more of it there is in that product.

Check out certain healthy-looking yoghurts that may be labelled 'low-fat' or 'fat-free' but are thickened and flavoured with heaps of sugar. Tinned soups, baked beans and most cereals contain sugar. Look for cereals with no added sugar in the health-food store or in the organic section of supermarkets.

Giving up sugar doesn't mean you have to stop eating sweet foods. Modern processing ensures that dried fruits like apricots, pears, dates, figs and prunes are now soft and juicy and, if you eat them straight from the freezer, they become deliciously chewy like toffee. Look for sugar-free yoghurts and desserts, and experiment with tinned fruit in natural juice and sugar-free jelly to make a fancy, fat-free trifle that even your kids will like.

Don't worry about the small amount of sugar in items like tomato ketchup or mayonnaise. The point of giving up refined sugar is because it encourages your body to store fat and causes cravings for more sugar. If you have some tomato ketchup with your meal, it is unlikely that you will finish the bottle! By the same token, if you are desperate for the occasional biscuit, the sugar-free ones made for diabetics are OK because they are sweetened with sorbitol. If, however, biscuits are a trigger food for you and you can't eat one without finishing the packet, then forget that idea (too much sorbitol causes diarrhoea).

Rule 2: All Main Meals Should Contain Protein

The main reason for eating protein at every meal is that it reacts with your body to get rid of your hunger and provide you with long-lasting energy. There is a certain hierarchy in the satiating effects of food. Protein is more satiating than carbohydrates – which are more satiating than fats. Your body is like an engine that runs continuously and needs constant fuel (food). It burns certain fuels immediately for energy and stores other types as fat.

Your body has almost no storage capacity for protein; therefore you can't eat too much at one go. Three steaks? A whole chicken? I don't think so. Your brain would send an urgent 'full up' message to your body and you would stop eating. This is actually how the Atkins Diet works. Forget the mumbo-jumbo. When you consume only protein to the exclusion of all other food, you automatically eat less.

Your body has a limited capacity for starchy carbohydrates like bread or pasta, but one large bowl of spaghetti carbonara is enough for most people. I know when you pass a bakery you can imagine yourself eating a whole loaf of crusty bread but could you really? Without butter? (I don't believe you.) Again, after a while, you would receive a 'full up' message from your hypothalamus – the part of the brain that controls appetite.

Sadly, however, your body has an almost unlimited capacity for storing fat – crisps, fries, nuts, chocolate, biscuits – and the signals from your brain are so weak that you can just over-ride them and continue eating.

Protein foods have something built into them that tells the hypothalamus when to signal 'stop eating'. Certain diet regimes encourage excessive amounts of protein with the exclusion of most other food groups. This could damage the kidneys if continued over a long period of time, but a 300-calorie portion of protein will make you feel fuller for longer than a carbohydrate meal containing the same number of calories.

Another reason for eating protein at every meal is that it stimulates the production of a hormone in the pancreas called glucagon, which counteracts the effects of insulin. Insulin is the fat-making hormone, remember, which floods into your bloodstream to regulate the amount of circulating glucose when you eat sugar or refined carbohydrates like white bread or potato. Eating more protein increases your levels of glucagon, which in turn lowers the amount of insulin circulating in your bloodstream.

Glucagon also affects your metabolic rate, which is the rate at which your body burns the food you eat as energy.

If your metabolism is high, you will use the food eaten immediately and not store much as fat. Conversely, if you have a slow metabolism, mainly through lack of exercise and eating haphazardly, you will store fat easily. Whereas insulin encourages your body to store fat, glucagon appears to shift your metabolism into fat-burning mode.

Eating oily fish like smoked salmon or mackerel raises the body's levels of the omega-3 essential fats that boost your brain power. Protein foods like turkey and chicken contain large amounts of the amino acids tryptophan and tyrosine, which raise the levels of the feel-good neurotransmitters serotonin and dopamine in your brain. Dopamine creates mental energy and alertness and increases your concentration. There is a lot of tyrosine in cheese, which is why you would have difficulty sleeping if you ate cheese last thing at night.

Another bonus is that protein foods protect your skin. Even if you use sun cream factor 240, some wrinkle-forming damage is bound to occur when you go out in the sun. Along with vitamin C, protein is the building block of collagen, the spongy substance that keeps skin looking firm and youthful, so eating protein foods can help protect you from getting lines and wrinkles.

Sugar, on the other hand, has just the opposite effect. The sugar molecules attach themselves to collagen, making the fibres stiff and inflexible, which accelerates the permanence of deep frown lines and nose-to-mouth creases.

According to Dr Nicholas Perricone, an American professor of dermatology, you can give yourself a nutritional facelift by eating fresh salmon three times a day. In his book, *The Perricone Prescription* (Thorsons), he claims that fish like salmon, mackerel and trout contain a chemical that stimulates nerve function and encourages the muscles under the skin to contract and tighten, smoothing out sags and bags (his expression).

'As protein is digested,' says Dr Perricone, 'it breaks down into amino acids that are used by the cells to repair themselves. Without adequate protein, our bodies enter into an accelerated ageing mode. Our muscles, organs, bones, cartilage, skin and the antibodies that guard us from disease are all made of protein. We cannot store protein in our bodies so we need to eat it three times a day.'

To sum up: protein food immediately gets rid of your hunger and raises your metabolic rate so that food gets burned up as energy rather than being stored as fat. Some protein foods like lamb and salmon are considered to be high in fat, but it is not necessarily this type of fat that has contributed to your problem – for that we can blame the fat you've been creating from sugar. Protein counteracts the harmful fat-storing insulin circulating in your bloodstream and encourages the production of the feel-good factors in your brain. Now you know why I recommend you eat protein at each meal.

Rule 3: Limit Starchy Carbohydrates

Carbohydrates, on the other hand, produce a calming effect on the body. That is why, when you feel stressed or anxious, you grab for stodgy carbs like bread and butter, pastries or cake, which have a soporific effect and diffuse any feelings of stress.

Carbohydrates are the main fuel your muscles need to work effectively, so a slow-release carb like porridge, sugar-free cereal or wholegrain bread at breakfast can set you up for the morning. You get double the benefit by combining these with protein, such as milk with cereal or eggs or cottage cheese with your toast. I don't really advise fruit juice in the morning – unless you like it for the taste. Fructose won't raise your blood sugar level or get your brain functioning.

I also don't advise the traditional cooked English breakfast of fried eggs, bacon and sausage. Your body doesn't crave fat in the mornings so a high-fat breakfast would just initiate a desire for more fat by signalling to the brain to make more of the fat-craving hormone, galanin. An omelette (one yolk, three whites) with grilled tomatoes and mushrooms, eaten with wholegrain toast, would be better.

After breakfast, don't have any more starchy carbs until later in the evening, if you fancy a snack. What you have for lunch will make a pivotal difference to the productivity of your afternoon. You want to stay alert and energized during the day, and a carb meal at lunchtime such as baked potato, sandwiches made with white bread or pasta will make you feel drowsy during the afternoon and in need of a sugary snack at tea time.

If you eat badly during the day, you lose control of the evening.

Just have protein with salad or vegetables at lunchtime, preferably not in a sandwich. I know it is convenient just to grab a sandwich, and the (usually) protein filling will slow down the absorption of the bread, but try staying off bread during the day for a while and see how it affects your energy levels – and your weight.

The best time to eat a carbohydrate snack is a couple of hours after your evening meal, which is usually the time people cast around for 'something sweet'. A planned snack such as a slice of toast with sugar-free jam, or a small bowl of cereal flakes mixed with a few sultanas, will satisfy any craving. Carbohydrates are calming and will ensure a good night's sleep.

If you don't normally eat anything after dinner, then leave it – that's fine. It's rather nice to know that you can if you want to. Just have your daily carb fix for breakfast.

When you come to the examples of how to plan your meals a few pages further on, you will see I suggest you have a carbohydrate-based evening meal once a week to prevent you getting bored. However, be careful what you choose: if something like pizza is a trigger food for you then select an alternative.

Rule 4: Fill up on Fruit and Vegetables

These are your main ally in weight loss – and health. If possible keep some fruit at work. Melon is very filling at any time and bananas come in their own handy packaging.

Most of the highly coloured salad vegetables, such as

carrots, peppers and tomatoes, contain a wide range of antioxidants. Great emphasis is now being placed on tomatoes because of the lycopene they contain, which has been proved to have a dramatic effect in reducing the incidence of cancer of the prostate. A report in the *Journal of Cancer* suggests there is an inverse association between ovarian cancer risk in pre-menopausal women and the amount of tomato lycopene they eat. A Swedish study has shown an apparent reduction of breast cancer in post-menopausal women whose diet included liberal portions of tomatoes.

Surprisingly, cooked tomato, tinned tomato and even tomato ketchup are all better sources of lycopene than raw tomatoes. So for optimum health, chop up some tomatoes in your salad, pop some under the grill to have with your evening meal and add tomato purée to your pasta sauce.

You can't eat healthily unless you have the correct foods in the house. Make sure your fridge is always packed with fresh fruit and vegetables. You know the ones you like – I don't have to tell you. The most popular vegetables are peas, sweetcorn, broccoli, cauliflower, Brussels sprouts, mangetout, asparagus, sweet potato, onions and carrots. Fresh peas in the pod make a satisfying nibble eaten raw, as does raw sweetcorn. I know these are considered to be starchy vegetables but the point of this eating plan is not to be too restrictive. Frozen veg is fine, though you can obviously live without items like fried onion rings.

Check out the 'Big Salad for Lunch' on page 119 for some more ideas.

As you increase your intake of vegetables, you may experience a slightly irritating, but temporary, symptom: wind. Journalist Maria McErlane, writing about her detox diet in *The Sunday Times Magazine*, confessed that she managed to clear an entire cinema by 'accidentally releasing such noxious fumes it could quite easily have been an Al-Qaeda attack'. Nothing as bad as that will happen to you, but as sugar tends to contribute to killing off the good bacteria in the bowel, giving up sugar and increasing your intake of vegetables is a way of naturally detoxifying your body. This may make you a bit windy for a while but it won't last very long.

You should eat foods that make you feel full. Fibrous foods like vegetables take a long time to digest. Most fat people eat very little fibre. If you try and control your weight without including fibrous foods, you will be fighting hunger all the time.

Rule 5: Have Regular, Small Meals throughout the Day

You have read this a million times in newspapers and diet books but do you do it? 'Haven't got time.' 'Can't be bothered.' 'I'm at work for God's sake!' Yeah, yeah, I hear you.

The main reason for eating at regular intervals is to keep your blood sugar level balanced. The most common reason for eating compulsively is hunger, so keeping your blood sugar level steady is probably the most important factor for being in control of your eating. If you allow yourself to get hungry, you think with your taste buds instead of your brain and often grab the nearest available snack, usually a chocolate bar or a bag of crisps. I want to forestall this by encouraging you to eat *before* you get hungry.

My advice is to glance at the clock when you have finished eating, count forward three hours and plan your next meal or snack at around that time. This is contrary to advice in other diet manuals where you are supposed to wait until you are hungry before you eat anything. Some diet writers advise you to ask yourself how hungry you are on a scale of 1 to 10 and not to eat until the need is compelling.

So how does that work? I can just imagine the scenario at Sunday lunch:

'Come on guys, lunch is ready, everyone sit down.'

'Not for me thanks, I'm not hungry right now.'

'But it's getting cold. When will you be hungry?'

'I don't know. My diet guru says I should only eat when I am very hungry, and I'm not at the moment.'

Two hours later you are stuck in a traffic jam and you are starving. So what do you do? Stop off at a newsagent, grab two chocolate bars, a packet of crisps and a coke and eat the lot in the car. That works!

Waiting until you are hungry does not work for me. I am a 'recovering' binger, and if you asked me whether I was hungry right now, my answer would probably be, 'I have no idea – I don't think so, but now that you mention it, I could fancy something.' I, along with most dieters, have lost the capacity to know whether my craving for food is actual hunger or in response to stress, hormones or just being fed up.

I also don't know when I am full – unless I am really stuffed. I cannot 'leave a little something on my plate' at the end of the meal. My binger's mentality protests, 'What's the point? I put the food on the plate, I am going to eat it – all of it!' I would rather control the size of portion than put food on the plate only to throw some away afterwards.

We eat for so many different reasons other than hunger – habit, social, boredom, seeing something we fancy, craving something someone else is eating – that to tell someone not to eat unless they are really hungry is wishful thinking. Very few people could do this. Possibly it is a way of 'getting in touch with your feelings' but by that time I would be 19 stone!

In my years of counselling overweight people, I have found that the best way to stay in control of your eating is to make sure you have something every three hours, even if it's just a drink or a few grapes. This means eating *before* the sensation in your stomach indicates hunger. This will keep your blood glucose level balanced, prevent you *getting* hungry, and keep your metabolic rate high.

Let's go back to the image of your body as a highly efficient fat-burning machine: you have to keep the engine stoked up with little bits of fuel (food) to keep it chugging along. If you let the engine get cold by allowing a long time to elapse between meals, your body is conditioned – as a result of thousands of years' evolution – to assume there is a famine. Being programmed for survival, it will slow down your metabolism to conserve your fat stores in case you are in danger of starving to death.

Your ancestors, of course, didn't have a Sainsbury's round the corner. When you do finally eat, the slower metabolism will ensure the food is stored as fat rather than used for immediate energy. This leads on to an understanding of why, if you try missing breakfast as an aid to weight loss, you lose out on two counts, nutritionally and metabolically. Your metabolism (engine) slows right down during the night. If you don't give it a nutritional kick-start in the morning, it will stay at a sluggish pace all day. **Hence: only fat people skip breakfast.**

Raising your metabolic rate by eating is called 'dietary-induced thermogenesis'. This increase is not influenced by the *amount* of food eaten as even a little bit of food will induce a measurable increase in energy expenditure. So make a commitment to eat something every three hours – and acknowledge that to achieve this, you have to *plan ahead*.

Decide what you are going to eat for the day: breakfast, mid-morning snack (or drink), lunch, mid-afternoon snack, dinner, possible evening snack. Every day for the first two weeks, write this down to make sure you stick to it. I know this sounds like a terribly boring thing to do, but it's only for two weeks so bear with it.

Jot it down *before* you embark on the day, not at the time of eating, so you can't change your mind when you feel vulnerable at tea time. You can always substitute one protein for another, such as tuna instead of chicken. If you plan to be away from home or away from a readily available supply of healthy foods, take a snack with you in your bag.

By following your own eating plan and knowing what you are going to eat at each meal, you will learn to separate your eating from your emotions. It will also relieve you of having to make decisions about what to eat during the day. This will prevent that 'What shall I have for lunch?' and, more importantly, that 'Shall I eat this or not?' confrontation when faced with temptation. If it is not on your eating plan for that day, then you don't eat it. No further discussion.

As you continue with this plan – one meal at a time, one day at a time – it gradually becomes a habit and you don't have to write it down any more. Just as you wake up in the morning and think, 'What shall I wear today?' so you will run though in your mind what you are going to eat that day for each meal. Do you need to take something out of the freezer for lunch? Will you be away from an available source of healthy food for more than three hours? If so, pack a snack.

Do not think further ahead than today. You can only live one day at a time and you don't want to evoke the 'Oh God, I can never have chocolate ever again' mindset. It is only for today: you are going to have this for breakfast; this for lunch; take an apple to eat on the train on your way home; and this for dinner. When it comes to tomorrow, you will decide tomorrow.

You will find this way of planning ahead the most helpful tool in gaining control of your eating. Don't dwell on the result – weight loss – just concentrate on eating healthy food *today* and the result will happen automatically.

Rule 6: Drink Extra Water

It is very irritating having to drink water if you are not thirsty. However, I have found with my clients that the ones who drink the water lose the weight. Don't ask me why – they just do. You have read how beneficial it is for your skin, your digestive system and your health to drink plenty of water, but few people remember to do it. The best way is to keep a bottle of water by your bed and take a swig when you wake up. I advise people to drink a full mug of water before each meal. The fact that you are going to put food into your mouth anyway should remind you to do it, and it does fill you up a bit so you are not tempted to eat until you feel stuffed.

I find that cold water is quite unpleasant to drink if you are not thirsty, but a splash of boiling water from the kettle takes the chill off it and makes it easier to get down. So come on, get into the habit of having eight big swallows of water before each meal. It might make you pee a bit more until your body gets used to it, but hey, think of all those toxins being flushed out. Cool.

Rule 7: Alcohol - Friend or Foe?

It is the most natural thing in the world to meet your friends for a drink, and there is no point in sitting there gazing miserably into a glass of water if you are accustomed to something stronger. The question of alcohol on a weight-loss plan is very subjective and, again, a matter of control. Alcoholic drinks have the same effect on the body as refined sugar, and if this affects your mood to the extent that it influences your choice of food, then I would advise you to cut it out.

Having said that, most of my clients seem able to enjoy a glass of wine with their evening meal to no ill effect. Others abstain during the week and allow themselves a small indulgence at weekends. Only you know what is right for you.

Some Meal Suggestions

The foods shown below are simply examples. You may choose entirely different ingredients and that's fine. As I said, I can't give you recipes because I have no idea what you like to eat. This is just to give you an idea.

On waking: a big swig of water – at least five big swallows. Keep a bottle by your bed.

Breakfast: (remember – only fat people skip breakfast)

> A big mug of water – eight big swallows – then either
> Sugar-free cereal with skimmed (or semi-skimmed) milk.

Or Porridge – sweeten with a big spoonful of sugar-free jam and/or Canderel/Equal or fructose.

Or Muesli base (from health-food shops) – add your own dried or fresh fruit and milk or yoghurt. Sweeten with Canderel/Equal or fructose.

Or Eggs with toast and low-fat spread.

Or Fruit salad and yoghurt. Couple of crispbreads.

Or Cottage cheese on toast and grilled tomatoes.

Mid Morning: tea or coffee with a piece of fruit (or not). If you are busy or not hungry at this time, you do not need to eat anything but plan to have lunch around 12.30 or 1pm – no later.

Lunch: remember that a carbohydrate meal – bread roll, sandwich, pasta, baked potato – at this time will make you sleepy during the afternoon and promote a sugar-craving around tea time.

> A big mug of water.
> Then some sort of protein – chicken, turkey, salmon, smoked salmon, prawns or ham with a large salad (*see 'Big Salad at Lunchtime', below*).

You shouldn't need anything else at this time. If you fancy 'something sweet' to finish a meal, have a couple of large dates or a small packet of raisins.

Mid Afternoon: remember that long gaps between meals cause your body to store fat. Make sure you eat something at this time, whether you are hungry or not.

Yoghurt and fruit (melon, grapes or a peach etc.).

Or   Cottage cheese and banana.

Or   A hard-boiled egg with some lettuce and a blob of mayo.

Or   A 30g (1 ounce) individual pack of low-fat cheese to nibble.

Or   2 strips of chicken breast with a tomato, carrot and cucumber.

See the end of this chapter for more snack ideas. If you do get hungry and there is nothing else available, have two rice cakes with sugar-free jam or a slice of 'rice-cheese' – from health-food shops. Rice cakes are the only carbohydrate permitted during the day, but treat as an 'emergency' food rather than the norm.

Evening Meal: remember – if you eat a lot of fat you will be fat. I am more concerned with the sugar content than the fat, but obviously slathering butter or oil on your food is not going to make you slim!

Large mug of water.

Then *either* (most evenings)

A large portion of protein and three or four different vegetables such as carrots, cauliflower, broccoli, sweet potatoes, Brussels sprouts, green beans, courgettes, peas, sweetcorn, asparagus. Use salad dressing as a dip to make the vegetables more interesting.

No carbs.

Or (once a week)

A carbohydrate-based meal like pasta (Bolognese sauce is fine; this plan is not about food combining) or baked potato or seafood risotto or pizza with salad or vegetables.

If you need dessert – such as fruit, dates, sugar-free jelly, yoghurt, flavoured dessert-mix made with skimmed milk etc. – have it later on in the evening when you may 'fancy' something instead of the carb snack below.

Later: do not go to bed hungry. If you feel niggly, have a small bowl of cereal or a slice of toast with a hot drink. This will make you feel calm and help you sleep.

If you are not in the habit of eating anything after your evening meal, then don't.

Big Salad at Lunchtime

Keep these basics in the fridge at all times:

Packet of mixed lettuce leaves
Tomatoes
Cucumber
Celery
Carrots, peeled and put in a bowl of cold water
Peppers – any colour – red are the sweetest
Chicory

Also keep a selection of vegetables for cooking, such as:

Asparagus
Cauliflower
Broccoli
Brussels sprouts
Green beans
Courgettes
Mangetout
For emergencies, tinned sweetcorn or asparagus and frozen
veg

You will need some sort of protein – about 115–170g (4–6oz) – such as:

Chicken
Turkey
Cottage cheese
Salmon
Smoked salmon
Smoked trout
Sardines or mackerel, tinned in brine
Tuna (small tin), tinned in brine
Hard-boiled eggs
Ham
Lean roast beef

★ Chop up the basic salad ingredients (grate the carrots)
and pile onto a plate. Make as much as you want.

★ Choose one or two other veg such as green beans and
cauliflower, cut them up and pop into the microwave for

a minute or two. Spoon on top of the salad. (Optional)

★ Cut up your chosen protein food and add to the salad.

★ Pour over some fat-free dressing. I tend to use quite a lot on my salad. My favourite flavour is honey mustard. Don't worry about the small amount of honey used in salad dressings as this is unlikely to set up a craving. There are lots of different varieties in the supermarkets. Experiment until you find one you like.

★ Mush it all up together and eat. Enjoy. Very healthy. Very filling. Should take ages to eat.

★ (No you don't need bread or crackers with it.)

For a change add:

★ A few olives, raisins or nuts – cashews, brazils, almonds.

★ A couple of spoonfuls of roasted root veg. Chop up red onions, parsnips, courgettes, sweet potatoes, put in a roasting pan (or foil pan so you can chuck the pan away afterwards), drizzle over a smidge of olive oil and roast for an hour. When cold, keep in the fridge. These vegetables will stay fresh for two or three days. They make a tasty addition to your salad, or have a few spoonfuls as a snack anytime.

★ Ready-made, shop-bought salads like beetroot or mixed bean salad. Pour off any oily dressing.

With this way of eating, you limit starchy carbohydrates to morning and, if needed, late evening (except for the occasional carb-based evening meal). This is to allow your body to utilize protein as energy and burn up your existing fat.

With the examples above, you will notice there is no mention of cakes, biscuits, chocolate, sweets, cheesecake or ice cream. If you can stay off sugary foods, you will be surprised how quickly you lose the taste for them – but you can only experience this for yourself.

I have not mentioned fruit juice because I feel this is just a way of ingesting loads of calories in three or four big gulps. It is much better to eat the whole fruit with the pleasure of chewing and swallowing, plus you get all the vitamins and fibre. I am also not keen on 'juicing' various combinations of fruit and vegetables for the same reason: a drink is not nearly as satisfying as a mini-meal of the same components. My clients have told me they quickly become irritated at having to dismantle and wash up the juicing machine after just one drink.

Milk

Do drink milk. So many women have cut out dairy food as part of a fad diet that they are seriously deficient in calcium – which can lead to bone problems later in life. Most dieters equate milk, cheese and yoghurt with injecting pounds of lard directly into their thighs. This is not the case, especially with low-fat varieties, and recent research has found the opposite effect.

According to Professor Michael Zemel of the University of Tennesee, writing in the *Journal of Nutrition*, dairy foods high in calcium can trick the body's metabolism into working overtime to lose weight. Zemel says, 'When your body is deprived of calcium in food, it begins conserving calcium. That mechanism prompts your body to produce higher levels of a hormone called calcitrol which then triggers a higher production of fat cells.'

Other clinical trials have found that getting enough calcium suppresses the production of calcitrol, and not only stimulates the body to burn more fat but also reduces the amount of new fat the body is capable of making. As Professor Zemel says, 'High levels of calcitrol "tell" fat cells to store themselves in the body and to expand. So, by eating too little dairy you are literally getting bigger, fatter fat cells. By eating more dairy foods you can make positive changes to your body-fat distribution by helping to shift calories from fat to lean body mass.' (I'm not quite sure what he means by that, but it sounds promising!)

You can get calcium from green vegetables, nuts, seeds and fish – especially the tinned variety with bones – but your body absorbs calcium from milk better than any other source. So pour skimmed or semi-skimmed (only 2 per cent fat) on your breakfast cereal, have some yoghurt with fruit at tea time, make your own frozen snack by liquidizing a ripe mango with some fat-free fromage frais, adding sweetener and pouring into ice-lolly moulds to keep in the freezer. Whip up some flavoured, sugar-free dessert with skimmed milk for your children's tea and have some yourself (if it doesn't 'start you off' – you know what I mean!).

Planning Ahead

🍌 **Put a banana in your car. Never leave home** 🍌
   without it.

To be successful with this plan, you must have the correct foods in the house. This means shopping at least twice a week for fruit and veg, and keeping a supply of protein foods in readily available portions in the freezer to add to your salad at lunchtime. It is easy to buy cooked chicken portions in supermarkets, as well as sliced ham, duck, chicken, roast beef and smoked trout or salmon. I buy ready-cut portions of fresh salmon – they usually come four to a pack – pop them under the grill for about five minutes each side and, when cold, wrap each one individually and keep in the freezer. Like me, you are unlikely to have this every day, so preparing two packs at a time should last you for weeks.

   Before you go to bed, take out a portion of something – chicken or salmon or whatever – and put it in the fridge to defrost overnight. This is what I mean by planning ahead. If you will be having lunch at work, it only takes a minute to put the salad ingredients – lettuce, tomato, cucumber, carrot, celery, red pepper, beetroot, sweetcorn – into a foil takeaway pack with a lid to take with you. You can use a plastic container but it means you have to lug it home with you and wash it. I find that in this throwaway age, the foil packs work better. Keep a bottle of your favourite salad dressing in your office – and some plastic forks.

You will also need to take an afternoon snack with you if you are working or will be away from home at this time. Fruit, yoghurt and cottage cheese are easily portable or available from local sources. If you are stuck then two thin, square rice cakes with a slice of 'rice cheese' in between is a tasty and easily portable snack wrapped in foil. This has become the emergency snack of many of my clients to eat on the bus, at the hairdresser's or in the car outside their children's school.

Reading the above it sounds like I expect you to leave home with a fully laden picnic basket each day. Not so. After the first couple of weeks, it becomes a habit to make up a little bag of food to take with you, and it is no bother at all. When tea time comes and you reach for your foil-pack of pineapple chunks and cottage cheese, you will be glad you made the effort.

Eating Out

Think 'fish 'n' veg' – your passport to health and slimness.

When eating out, think 'fish and veg', whether it's lunchtime or in the evening. Yes, I realize that eating in nice restaurants is meant to be a pleasure and no-one is preventing you from trying new dishes and enjoying your old favourites. However, if you are unsure, the 'fish and veg' rule is a good one to bear in mind. You are well aware of which foods are fattening, and during your initial weight-loss period you need to make wise food choices at all times. You can't control the amount of fat in a restaurant-cooked meal but you can avoid the obvious choices of fried foods and thick sauces.

Olive oil is fattening. Believe it. So many clients have told me defiantly, 'Olive oil is supposed to be good for you'. And? It's still fattening. Olive oil does contain the fat-soluble vitamins A, D, E and F, but so does every other kind of fat. Olive oil manufacturers do seem to employ better PR people than other oil producers but it is still 100 per cent fat. Use it with caution.

Living Slim

I call this eating plan 'Living Slim' because that is exactly what it is. This is not a 'diet' in which, once you stop the plan, all the weight goes back on. There is not a 'weight-loss' phase then a 'maintenance' phase. As you get into this method, you will gradually build what I call an 'eating blueprint' that is exclusive to you. Day by day you will get used to thinking ahead of where you will be during the day and what food you will be eating.

Eating is a habit. Most people eat the foods they are

used to eating at the times they are used to eating them. If you are used to 'something sweet' after a meal, you don't have to deprive yourself, but use something non-addictive like dried fruits, a sugar-free biscuit or a yoghurt.

Living Slim is a commitment that only you can make. We've already agreed that gimmicky diets don't work for you. A personal eating plan designed by you, for you, based on healthy food choices that you can live with day by day does work. For bingers, this is a way of staying in control of your eating, by planning ahead and knowing what you are going to eat at each meal. This is far better than mindless eating where you wait until the mealtime is upon you, then make choices based on whatever is available – usually accompanied by bread or fries.

Eating by the clock also eliminates the compulsive need to 'stuff it all in now'. You know you are going to eat in two hours anyway, so you tell yourself to wait till then.

You will find that getting into a habit of eating healthy food at regular hours day by day will be an enormous help when the inevitable 'plateau' strikes, usually five or six weeks into your plan. This is when your weight-loss appears to come to an abrupt halt and the number on the scales resolutely refuses to budge. We look at this in more detail in Chapter 8.

Dealing with Temptation

☺   **A craving is only a thought, a feeling. It will pass.**   ☺

It is impossible to go through life and not, occasionally, be faced with a tempting selection of fattening food, either on holiday, in a restaurant or at a party. In making your food choices, you have to decide what is more important – eating the fattening food or being slim. You can't do both – not even 'just this once'. You have tried. It doesn't work if 'just this once' triggers a binge.

There are some people who can break off two squares of chocolate and put the rest of the bar back. They are in control of their eating and are probably male, married to me or naturally slim (and not likely to be reading this book!). If how you look, how you feel and your level of energy is important to you, then make the commitment to cut out sugar and eat healthily.

Will it be for ever? No, of course not. It is asking too much for anyone never to eat fattening food ever again. The important thing is to be in control of your eating, and this is what we are working towards here. Once you have lost the amount of weight you want and have sta-bilized at your desired weight for at least three months (read the last few words again), you may choose to indulge in a fattening treat that you wouldn't eat in the course of a normal day. This could be a slice of cake at a friend's house or a wicked dessert at a special restaurant – but this is only eaten *on a particular occasion*.

In other words, you would give yourself permission to have that one thing – even if you have two or three slices – and enjoy it without feeling guilty or that you have 'broken your diet so you might as well go on eating for the rest of the night and (all together now) start again tomorrow'. That is the old way of thinking, the always-on-a-diet way. Making a conscious decision to indulge on a particular occasion simply means you eat, you enjoy and you stop eating when you have finished. You do not then cast around for other fattening things to eat. This is being in control of your eating and is the exact opposite to the 'Oh sod it!' response, which is the precursor of a binge.

The following day you go back to your normal eating blueprint, knowing that it is not one meal that makes you fat, but what you eat on a day-by-day basis that determines how you look and feel. You may look in your diary and see a birthday party coming up in a few weeks and decide to have some cake on that occasion. This way of thinking allows you to stay in control rather than *being* controlled by food. Does that make you feel better?

However, if these fattening treats happen every week, they will soon begin to happen every day – and you will be back to square one. Choose your fattening treat days carefully and have at least four clear weeks between each one.

Having a definite plan of eating soon becomes a way of life, rather than a temporary solution. Making healthy food choices is a positive action rather than the deprivation of being on a diet. Eliminating refined sugar from your diet will give you energy both mentally and physically, and each day you do it makes the following day easier.

In this way, you are living like a slim person.

Snack Ideas and Food Tips

★ Lettuce Roll-up. Choose a large, flat lettuce leaf and place on it a slice of smoked salmon, a few cucumber strips down the middle, a blob of mayonnaise and roll it up as you would do a Chinese pancake. Have two of these as an afternoon snack. You could substitute a slice of ham and a blob of mustard if you wish.

★ From-frais Dip. Tip half a large pot of fat-free fromage frais into a bowl. Stir in a third of a bottle of oil-free dressing, and Canderel/Equal to taste. This is delicious with raw or cooked veg and is completely fat-free. Will last several days in the fridge.

★ A big mug of thick veggie soup is a great filling snack. Take it to work in a flask or buy from Pret A Manger or a sandwich shop.

★ Most supermarkets sell portions of ready-made fruit salad - delicious with vanilla yoghurt poured on top.

★ For a more substantial snack, eat one roast chicken drumstick at tea time. Wouldn't dream of it! Why not?

★ From Gillian, a former client: mash a small banana in a bowl, stir in 10 almonds and a few raisins. Eat with a teaspoon. Everyone likes baby food.

★ Two sticks of celery stuffed with low-fat soft cheese and 4 dates. This will give you the crunch and the sweetness.

★ In a rush? Have a small tin of sugar-free baked beans, eaten with a teaspoon out the tin.

★ Cut an apple into quarters, then into eighths. Eat by dipping each piece into sugar-free toffee yoghurt.

★ Ten walnuts eaten with a small packet of raisins and triangle of light cheese spread.

★ Desperate for a sweetie? Try the little packs of sugar-free sweets sold in every chemist and newsagent in lots of different flavours. These are sweets you can suck quite happily without rotting your teeth.

★ For your evening meal, try Bolognese sauce poured over lightly cooked, shredded cabbage. Who said 'yuck!'? Pour it over 'corn pasta' then.

★ Nice dessert: large Bramley apple, whole and unpeeled. Remove the core and score round the circumference of the apple with the tip of a knife to just break the skin. This will stop it exploding all over your oven. Fill the middle aperture with a mixture of sultanas and sugar-free jam. Put the apple into a shallow glass bowl with some water and a bit more jam to make a sauce, sprinkle with fructose and bake in a moderate oven (180°C/350°F/Gas Mark 4) for an hour.

★ Good tip: to keep a packet of lettuce fresh, cut along the top of the packet. Stuff a sheet of kitchen roll down each side to catch the condensation. Fold over the top of the packet and secure with tape. Change the sheet of kitchen roll each time you use some of the lettuce. It will now stay fresh for several days.

⊛ Chewing gum signals to your stomach to ⊛ expect food. When that doesn't happen, it sets up a craving. Therefore, chewing gum makes you hungry.

Conversation with Client, Barbara, aged 56

B: *I'm not really sure how this diet works. I expected you to give me a diet sheet or something – or at least a list of calorie-counted foods – but you are saying I can eat more or less whatever I want provided I stay off sugar. I find this quite strange as I am used to counting points or fat units, but you don't seem to think this is necessary. So how am I meant to lose weight? I don't understand.*

Me: *What part of 'Don't eat sugar' don't you understand?*

B: *But surely it's much harder to shift the weight at my age. I am menopausal and naturally I have put on a lot of weight round my middle, which looks awful. I hate having to buy clothes with elasticated waists. I'm told that as you get older your metabolism slows down, making it even more difficult to lose weight. Also we eat out a lot, and entertain friends at home, so there is always tempting food around. All my friends are struggling as well. It's really hard.*

Me: *And your point is…?*

Conversation with Client

C: *Can I have potato salad or coleslaw on my lunchtime salad?*

Me: *It's better not to have potato salad because that's a starchy carb which is preferable to avoid during the day, but a spoonful of coleslaw won't hurt. I know that it is drenched in mayo but you don't have to be so pedantic. As long as you are cutting out the obvious sugary stuff, feel free to eat everything else.*

C: *You haven't mentioned anything about portion sizes. How much chicken could I eat?*

Me: *You know what a portion size looks like. Obviously, a chicken breast or leg portion is the norm, but I don't want you to get hung up on this and start measuring and weighing. Just eat and enjoy.*

C: *What about breakfast? You say it's OK to have carbs then so can I have cereal and toast?*

Me: *Do you need both? A bowl of cereal with milk and some sultanas in it should be enough to see you through the morning. If you are hungry mid-morning, have some fruit or a yoghurt then. It's better to spread out your food intake rather than eat a lot in one go, except for vegetables when you can have as much as you like.*

C: *I found this organic cereal called Millet Rice Flakes that I've been having for breakfast. How much should I have?*

Me: *Put your hand in the packet and however much cereal you can pull out clutched in your fist, that's what you put in the bowl.*

C: *Fair enough. Would I use the same measuring device for porridge?*

Me: *You could do I suppose.*

C: *Before or after it's cooked?*

Chapter Five

You Either Get it – or You Don't

Here's one to think about:

'Life is a rip-off when you expect to get what you want. Life works when you choose what you've got. Actually, what you've got is what you chose. To move on, choose it.' – Werner Erhard, creator of Erhard Seminars Training (est)

When someone tells you a joke and you laugh, that means you 'get it'. You don't 'understand' a joke; you 'get it'. If someone has to explain the punch line, it isn't funny any more.

So, *get this*: if you want to be slim there is no point in eating the sort of food that makes you fat. No, not 'obviously'. Many people can't seem to make the connection between their shape and what they put into their mouths.

Are You in Denial?

'I'll just have **one** little taste' – **don't** lie to yourself.

I was at a wedding reception watching a plump lady chatting with a group of friends and eating canapés one after the other. As each tray came by, she reached out and selected something from the array of mini-pizzas, sausage rolls, mushroom vol-au-vents and goujons, and stood there munching happily. Later, she was at my table and asked me why I wasn't having any dessert. I replied that I was too full after the first three courses, which was both true and my usual excuse for not eating sugar (I never go into detailed explanations). She said she wished she could be so disciplined; she was on a strict diet but somehow just couldn't lose weight. I stopped myself saying, 'But you ate about 2,000 calories before you even sat down for dinner, you silly cow!' – I just sympathized and agreed that it was very hard.

Other people have told me that they really work hard at staying slim, and in the next breath explain that you can't expect to stick to a diet on holiday. Besides, if you are on a cruise 'it's all paid for' so it's a shame not to eat it. Oh well, there's your passport to Fatsville. By all means eat it – it's your choice – but don't kid yourself you want to be slim.

A client told me she couldn't understand why her weight was creeping up and up. She explained that she never had any high-fat food in the house like cheese or creamy desserts except when she entertained. On these occasions she had to eat to keep her guests company – but that was only twice a month. She had obviously forgotten to tell her body to opt out of storing fat while she spent the week following a dinner party finishing up the leftovers.

Is it me or do these people genuinely exist in a state of denial? Here's another example: I was at a small dinner party recently and the lady sitting next to the hostess refused the luscious-looking chocolate gateau because she was on Weight Watchers. After finishing her alternative choice, fruit salad, she picked up a knife and said, 'I'm just going to have a tiny taste, but let me cut it,' and sliced off a thin sliver of gateau, saying, 'That's only about four points.' A few minutes later she did it again – and again. Then she had to 'tidy it up'. By the time we left the table she had eaten the equivalent of two huge slices of fat-laden, creamy gunge. Lady, you just don't get it!

I've seen this phenomenon over and over again in people. This sense of 'disconnection' between what we eat and how fat we are seems to be universal.

Exercise Denial

I see a similar disconnection when it comes to exercise. Another 40-something woman I met insisted to me that exercise didn't work. She went to the gym three times a week, she said, but it made no difference at all to her shape. A colleague who works at that health club told me that this lady comes along and perches on the stationary bike, pedalling languidly for as long as it takes her to flick through *Hello!* magazine. Sometimes she comes with her friend, both in designer tracksuits, full make-up and jewellery. They stroll for 10 minutes on adjacent treadmills, chatting all the time, then sit for a further hour drinking full-cream cappuccinos in the café while eyeing up the tennis coach.

They don't get it! But you are now beginning to, aren't you…?

Why Do You Overeat?

◌ **Look** back over the years. It is the same foods, ◌ the same patterns, the same excuses.

While these thoughts crystallize in your mind, you should also get this: as far as your food intake is concerned, it's not *what* you eat or *how often* but *why*. Why do you overeat and why is it always biscuits, chocolate, crisps, cakes, ice cream, etc.?

That is the reason you don't lose weight on a diet – or if you do, why you put the whole lot back on again. It is because you haven't figured out the *cause* of your overeating. Until you do and you can put it behind you, you will never be able to lose weight and keep it off. Think about it: if a significant part of how you live right now involves regular, or even sporadic, comfort eating on high-fat carbs – let's call this Lifestyle A – and you put yourself on a diet where you can only eat meat and lettuce – Lifestyle B – then it stands to reason that within a short period you will return to Lifestyle A. That is how you have always lived. It's what you know and what you are comfortable with, even if ultimately you aren't comfortable with the results.

Are You Addicted to Food?

You have to treat the source of your eating disorder because your overeating is a symptom of this disease.

Being addicted to food is the same as any other addiction such as to nicotine or alcohol. Out of all the addictive substances, food is the only one from which you cannot totally abstain. The alcohol treatment failure rate is 85 per cent, and that is a substance you never have to touch again for the rest of your life.

Although some experts claim that addiction is an inherited trait, the evidence from studies of twins and adopted children is far from clear. If genetics were behind all of our actions, then behaviour patterns, eating patterns and body shapes would be the same as our parents and would be fully predictable. While genes may be implicated in some cases, the key to adult behaviours and attitudes is usually childhood experiences, the main contributory factor being parental care. So even if there is such a thing as a predetermined genetic vulnerability, your childhood history may determine whether or not you will succumb to it.

The Link with Childhood Experiences

When I refer to childhood experiences, I am not talking about severe maltreatment. To be addicted to food you don't have to have been beaten, abused or emotionally neglected as a child. Clearly, however, those are terrible experiences and could be significant triggers for problems in later life. There is evidence that some children who suffer sexual abuse go on to develop eating disorders: girls in particular might overeat significantly in order to make themselves deliberately fat and therefore less attractive to men. Other girls might become anorexic in order to delay the onset of puberty so they don't have to see themselves as 'sexual beings'. It's terribly sad, but thankfully it is not widespread, and it certainly doesn't apply in reverse: there is no suggestion that eating disorders mean any kind of child abuse. The reasons for our problems with food are many and various and we need to get to the root of *yours*.

Maybe you just didn't get the love and attention you wanted as a small child, so your need to be fed and cuddled wasn't met. Maybe your parents separated or divorced, leaving you with a residual niggling guilt that you were to blame, that you caused the parent to leave because you were naughty or you weren't worthy or lovable enough for them to stay. Children are notoriously self-centred and think everything that happens in their little world must have something to do with them.

Depending on their age, children will respond to these feelings in a number of ways. Maybe they understood what was going on, or maybe it was just a sense of unease, of insecurity, of general unhappiness. It may not have been at home – the bad experiences could well have been at school or interacting with other children – but children might lack the language, the simple word power, to explain to their parents what is happening.

Whatever negative feelings you experienced, they don't just fade away in later life. We comfort ourselves in the ways we learned as a baby. Eating yourself into a bloated stupor becomes a way of stemming the hurt, a totally reliable antidepressant substitute for mother's milk, for which you do not have to be kept waiting because it is self-administered on demand.

When did you start overeating or having problems with food? When did you begin to use food as a comfort mechanism? You might need to think about this in some considerable depth, going back to your childhood if necessary. Let's face it: when you were two years old, you may have had temper tantrums out of frustration, but you didn't then go and raid the fridge or grab some peanut butter and eat it straight from the jar with a knife! *Something* started this habit for you.

In my own case it was when I was six years old and my mother, for reasons best known to herself, sent me away to a boarding school, 300 miles from our home in Maidenhead. The youngest pupil in the whole school, I was desperately lost, lonely and unhappy. I remember wandering around the building feeling bewildered and terrified of the hordes of 'big' girls (who must have been all of nine or ten) rushing all around me. I was there for nearly two years and my memory is of being unhappy and fearful most of the time. My only solace was the tuck box, which each child brought from home, filled with sweets and chocolate. We were allowed to take one small ration a day but I filled my pockets and hid them under my pillow so that I could lie in bed at night and eat my way solidly through them.

In later years when I asked my mother why she sent me away, she made vague references to the difficulties they all experienced after the war, but the war had been over a long time by then. My parents were in the throes of moving to a house in north London, and I think she just wanted me out of the way so she could get on with sorting out the building and decorating. Whatever the reason, that was the start of my childhood habit of secreting sweet food in hiding places and bingeing on it later when no-one was looking – a pattern of behaviour that was to characterize much of my adult life.

The resentment against my mother lasted many decades, as did the bingeing. Eventually, however, I matured enough to realize that she simply did what she thought was best at the time, and that in those days no-one was clued-up enough to recognize the obvious behavioural signs of distress I was exhibiting at the school and take me away. I forgave my mother – and no, it wasn't an instant process, it took some years – but once I managed to stop blaming her for my distorted eating habits, the resentment eventually turned to love. I realized that I was now an adult and responsible for my own life and I had to 'let go' of my past so that I could control my future – and my eating.

Identifying Your Trigger

What, then, was *your* trigger? What happened in your past that prompted you to start grabbing for food when you were under stress, or simply bored? What bad experience made you start eating to push it away? Sometimes you start doing something for one reason and continue doing it for another. You reacted to a challenge or a stressful occurrence by eating a large amount of stodgy food, so the next time you were faced with a similar challenge, you repeated this same action until it got to be a habit.

Next, you have to establish what satisfaction you are getting from your comfort eating. You must be getting a benefit from this or you wouldn't keep doing it. I know that will sound peculiar in the context of overeating but stick with me here: there has to be a subconscious reward in there, or a comfort, some kind of 'payoff', or you simply would not continue doing it. If you burn your hand taking a hot dish straight from the microwave, next time you use an oven glove. You learn pretty fast the things that don't work and don't repeat them. So your comfort eating must be working for you on some level or you would stop. Maybe you hate the result but that has not, so far, persuaded you to behave differently. There has to be a reason.

I've taken many clients through this process. Their answers are often: 'It's a relief', 'As soon as I start eating I feel calmer', 'I know it's going to make me fatter but right at that moment, I just don't care' – or as one lovely lady put it, 'When I'm lonely, it's like having a party in my mouth'!

For many women in particular, this allows them to perpetuate the fantasy that if their shape were different, everything else in their lives would be different too. If they had a perfect body they would have a man, a well-paid job and high self-esteem too. Their fat literally becomes a barrier to reality. By staying fat they don't have to confront whatever fears of power, intimacy, rejection, sexuality or success are coming between them and their dream world.

We're all in this together, folks! No-one gets to adulthood without experiencing distressing events and occasionally having bad things happen to them. This is called growing up, I believe... and we all coped with it in different ways. Something along the way pulled you up and caused you to start eating too much, either continually or as a response to particular situations. Whatever, or whoever, was responsible, the best thing about it is that it's over. It's in the past and you can make the decision that you will no longer be held hostage by that event – or that person – for one more minute. You have a different life now; you are an adult and you are going to move on. You no longer need to block things out with food.

Get this: no diet programme will take away the 'need' if you use food as a coping mechanism. If you're using it for a reason other than nutrition, you need to confront that reason or put something in its place. Otherwise you will always go back to it. Once you experience that 'mind shift' where you look at yourself squarely in the mirror and say 'I do not have to do this any more' – that is the moment your weight will start to go, forever.

Defiantly Fat

Sometimes you have to take action even if you don't want to. One of my clients, who was sent to me by her doctor, tipped the scales at nearly 19 stone. She said, 'I know I'm overweight but it's been creeping up over the years and I've got used to being big. I'm on the Fatkins diet. I just want to eat the foods I enjoy eating. I don't like salad and I've never liked fruit. I hate exercise; it's sweaty and boring. I can't be bothered to cook; it's much easier to get takeaways and the kids prefer it anyway. Yet my doctor is concerned that my blood pressure is high and I get breathless going up the stairs. He says that I am a prime candidate for Type 2 diabetes and possibly worse!'

Lady, you are not getting it here! You have two teenage boys and you are brushing aside the fact that your doctor is worried about your health. Experts from Cancer Research UK say that women who are obese are 60 per cent more likely to die from breast cancer because of hormonal changes, and more than twice as likely to die from cancer of the womb or gullet. Diagnosis of the disease may be delayed because of body size. Professor Julian Peto, of the Institute of Cancer Research, said, 'English people are getting fatter and it is causing cancer. Being overweight is the most avoidable cause of cancer in non-smokers.'

As I said, sometimes you just have to do things you don't like. No-one likes paying taxes but you have to. Looking after your health is part of being grown-up, especially if you have other people relying on you and who love you. You have to take care of yourself before you can take care of others.

Children react differently. If you say to a child, 'Eat your cauliflower,' the child will say, 'I hate cauliflower. Why should I eat something I don't like?' For a child this makes perfect sense. For you, as an adult, eating cauliflower and other vegetables is part of a plan to keep your weight down and keep you healthy. Immaturity means short-term reward because the payoff of slimness and vitality seems so remote. Grow up and do whatever is necessary for your long-term health. You won't win if you feel resentment because of the adjustments you have to make for the sake of your health. Get over it.

Changing for the Better

If your life is going to get better, it will be *because you make it better*. Analyse what isn't working so that you can make the necessary changes to get it to work. You can't change a situation if you don't acknowledge that there is something that needs to change. Is your job particularly stressful? Do you seem to be taking on more responsibility than you can comfortably deal with? If you work for other people, do your bosses expect more of you than you feel you can produce?

What about your home life? Dealing with children –big or small – always seems to involve food. Can you get help or teach them to do more for themselves? Even young children are open to negotiation, particularly if there is a reward involved. Other stresses mentioned by clients are relationships with parents, particularly those who are elderly or infirm, tensions within the family, holidays and just plain exhaustion. People will use you if you let them. Don't let them.

Obviously you can't just chuck in your job or put your children into care – however tempting – but you can make behavioural changes, such as eating sensibly and no longer using the stress in your life as an excuse to overeat. Feelings pass, moods change, things will get resolved – or not. Don't hand over your feelings to food, thereby inducing other feelings when the results of the food become apparent.

It's up to You

☺ **Don't start any sentence with the words 'I can't'.** ☺

You know and experience everything that happens through your own perceptions. Only you can determine how you feel. Other people can create an event or behaviour that you have to react to, but it is up to you how you choose to feel about them.

You are in control of your body. It is yours, you own in, you live in it. If past choices have made that body fatter than you would like, decide to make difference choices. The rest of this year will go by whether you start to do something about improving your life or not. So start now. You can't keep repeating the same actions and expect to get different results. Make a plan and stick to that plan. You only have one life.

The most important person in your life is you. Does that sound selfish? Women are notorious for putting their family members first and themselves last. But when you think about it, if you are not as fit and healthy as you can be, you are depriving these important people in your life by not giving them the best 'you' that you can. If you are always tired, grumpy or hating yourself and the way you look, how do you think that reflects on your family? Would you enjoy being around *you*? Would *you* look forward to spending time with *you* as you are today? Surely your family and friends deserve the happy, slim, energetic person that is in you somewhere – don't they?

Decide what you want then consider what you are willing to exchange to get it. Successful people are simply those who make better decisions. Success doesn't just happen by chance; it's a decision. Either do it or don't. 'I'll try' isn't a commitment.

Get this: you can't eat fattening food and still be slim. Some people can. You can't. Tough!

Dealing with 'Deprivation'

☪ **Don't say 'I can't eat chocolate'. You *can*** ☪
eat chocolate. You just choose not to.

People trying to lose weight always attempt to factor fattening foods into their daily diets by awarding a number of points to them or calling them 'sins' or 'my afternoon treat'. Well, your afternoon treat is keeping you fat and continuously reactivating your craving for sugar. That doesn't mean you can't have an afternoon snack; it means choosing one that is healthier and more satisfying that the momentary cloying taste of a chocolate-coated biscuit.

Can't bear the thought of going through life without chocolate? If by 'through life' you mean on a daily basis, then fine, eat it, but don't kid yourself that you want to be slim. 'But I would feel *deprived* if I had to give up choco-late' is the next whinge. Don't even suggest that you are deprived. People living in the developing world with no access to clean water or shelter are deprived. People who have no choice but to sleep on the streets are deprived. *You* are not deprived because you decide to go through the day without shoving a chocolate brownie into your face!

Get this: deprivation is a big nutritional lie that people have been led to believe for years; that if you can't have your favourite fattening food every day, life is just not worth living. The fact that this particular food is doing the most terrible harm to your shape, your health and your self-esteem doesn't seem to register.

If you are someone who habitually turns to food for comfort and can't stop eating until you feel nauseous, dep-rivation isn't about whether you can eat chocolate or not. For you, and people like you, deprivation is feeling fat and lumpy, hating yourself, not being able to wear the clothes you want and feeling that your whole life is out of con-trol. And all for the transient taste of something sweet.

Suppose you were allergic to nuts. You know that if you ate nuts, your throat would swell up and you could die. So you don't eat them and have no sense of deprivation in this regard. It is the same with sugar. Obviously you won't die from eating some sugar, but it can certainly make your thighs swell up and lead to you feeling bloated, fat and miserable.

It is simply a matter of changing the way you think. You can think, 'Oh dear, I can't eat chocolate because I am on a diet but I do miss it' – or you can think 'I *can* eat chocolate, I can eat anything I like, but I *choose* not to eat it because I know it makes me fat, depressed and perpetuates a craving for more chocolate. It is not a problem.' This is free choice, not deprivation.

When you tell yourself you'll be deprived, you create stress in your mind because of your doubt and uncertainty as to whether you will be able to do this. But life without sugar is infinitely more enjoyable, as you will discover for yourself.

Making Realistic Choices

You may well be thinking that surely it should be possible to incorporate all foods into your diet in moderation. It should – but wishful thinking and reality are two different concepts. You are and always have been trying to incorporate fattening foods into your diet – so you tell me: how does that work for you? Do you have the shape you want or are you still struggling? If you continue to try and control a substance like sugar, which produces an addictive reaction in your body, you will be fighting a food battle in your mind every day. 'Shall I eat this or not?' 'Am I having a "good" day or a "bad" day?' 'If I eat this now, I won't have anything later'. And on it goes.

Immediate gratification, however small, is more powerful than some remote reward. This is why people smoke, take drugs and overeat. By nature we are impulse-driven and immature, wanting whatever we want now, even though the long-term penalty may be obesity, ill health or worse. This may be human nature but *you don't have to buy into it.*

Get this: if there is a substance you can't control, then that substance is controlling you. Stop being reactive. Stop giving in to the marketing machine. Why is there junk food around? *Because you are buying it and eating it.* Those adverts will suck you in if you let them. You don't have to do it. Get it into your head that instant gratification is childish and harmful to the way you function on a daily basis. Learn to control those impulses. Alternatively, stay fat. It really doesn't matter in the grand scheme of things – whatever you decide is unlikely to be on the news tonight, because it only matters to you.

🍓 **If you don't buy it, you won't eat it.** 🍓

It is your choice. Which is more important to you: living like a slim person, or continuing to fight your craving for fattening food and whingeing about your weight? You can't do both. You have tried that for long enough to know that it doesn't work. Time for a rethink, perhaps?

On the television programme, *The Fat Club*, several participants, including politician Ann Widdecombe, lost an appreciable amount of weight over a six-month period. This was conducted under the relentless eye of the television camera and a hard-nosed trainer who attempted to bully them into submission. After the graduation, they all got together to celebrate their weight loss – with a slap-up meal complete with wine and creamy desserts. They just don't get it!

Make the Commitment

It is fine to dream of being slim, fit and vibrant but what you really need is a goal. In the dream you focus only on where you want to be; the difference with a goal is that you work out how you're going to get there. The first step is to make the commitment that you are not going to be fat any more. This doesn't have to be a big deal. All you have to do is to decide to put only healthy food into your body, cut out the junk food and follow the suggestions for 'Living Slim' outlined in the last chapter.

Formulate a Plan

★ Make a plan that fits in with your personal lifestyle and stick to it. Identify the high-risk times during each day

when you go for sugary food, and work out a strategy
to deal with them by avoiding areas of temptation or
substituting healthier snacks. Turn up to meetings *after*
your colleagues have finished the Danish pastries.

★ Clear the decks. If a situation is bothering you, take
the necessary steps to change it, which means finding a
way of dealing with it that doesn't involve food. Feeding
a problem with food just pushes it out of sight and
doesn't achieve anything.

★ If you need to confront someone, think it through and
do it. Emotional upsets happen and often blow over.
Whatever the outcome, you will be better equipped to
deal with the consequences if you have not stuffed
yourself with junk food.

★ If there is a situation you can't change, that you need
to live with on a daily basis, then you need to formulate
a plan to 'manage' it. Can you arrange to put some
space between yourself and whatever is bothering you
- even for an hour or so? A walk in the sunshine, a rest
listening to music for a while can change your brain
chemistry from jagged to calm.

Have a Specific Strategy

Constantly reinforce the thought that you are not going
to be fat any more. The first step is to make the necessary alterations to your surroundings and lifestyle.

★ Make your kitchen 'safe'. That means banishing any

food that has started you off on a binge in the past. If
you 'need' to have biscuits in the house, buy ones you
don't particularly like (come on now, there must be
some!) and hide them in a top cupboard, making whoever
'has' to have them climb up and get them.

★ Make your desk safe. You know what to keep in there
for emergencies: only items of the headache tablet and
tampon variety, nothing edible.

★ Plan ahead. Plan what you are going to eat at each meal
or snack-time during the day. Write it down for the
first two weeks and stick to it.

★ Don't go on a crash diet to 'give you a head start'.

★ Don't skip meals.

★ Don't indulge in compulsive eating. Eat every three
hours to prevent hunger and help you through your
high-risk times.

★ Sling out any clothes that have expandable waists and
anything baggy or saggy – accept that you buy these
so you can hide in them. Once you lose weight you will
not need your 'fat clothes' any more. This time there is
no going back.

Be Realistic

When food was less plentiful, fat symbolized riches
and prosperity. Wealthy people were able to afford more
food than poor people. Today, in the West, thinness is
emblematic of having so much that one can choose to
do without. Queen Victoria was proud to be plump. The

Duchess of York is a spokesperson for Weight Watchers.

Any woman who says she hates her body is expressing more than a wish to be slim. It's extremely difficult
for us to separate ourselves from our cultural standards.
The body shapes we admire reflect the taste of our
times. Today, clothes are designed for slim people. This
makes life particularly painful for those whose shape is
not currently in vogue (or in *Vogue* magazine).

Women are in an impossible position today: they have
to be sexy and desirable wives, nurturing, hands-on
mummies, high-powered wage earners and *slim*. Being
slim sends a visual message to the world that a woman is
competent, attractive, disciplined, efficient and in control
of herself.

You do not have to buy into this. Many dieters model
themselves on an unrealistic ideal. For most people, achiev-
ing the body weight and shape presented in the media is
not a reasonable, appropriate or achievable goal. Logically
you know this; you know that models probably exist on
three square vomits a day. Maybe your eating patterns and
yo-yoing weight symbolize, on one hand, your unwilling-
ness to accept a cultural indictment that, on another level,
you have internalized as an ideal. You want to be slim – and
that's it. But how slim? What shape do you want to be?

The Body Mass Index

The global gauge for assessing weight is the Body Mass
Index (BMI). You calculate your BMI by dividing your

weight in kilograms by your height in metres squared. If you weigh 10 stone (63.6kg) and are 5ft 8in tall (1.73m), that's 63.6 divided by 1.73 squared ($1.73 \times 1.73 = 2.99$), which comes to 21.2 – which is just right. A BMI of less than 18.5 is regarded as underweight, the normal range being 18.5 to 24.9. Anyone with a BMI over 25 is considered overweight and those above 30 are classified as obese.

An easier way to decide if you're too fat is if your jeans won't do up.

There's no Hurry

Let's get real here. You know that it took time to accumulate the flab and it will take time for it to go. Accept a realistic goal weight that is right for your personal figure and age. If you haven't been 8 stone since you were 15, you are not going to get down and stay there. Instead of choosing a specific weight, decide on a weight that you can stay *just under*. If you would like to weigh around 9 stone, then aim to stay *under* 9.4. This allows for the natural fluctuations that occur with every woman due to water retention, hormones or Cadbury's Creme Eggs.

It doesn't matter how slowly the scales go down as long as they are going in the right direction. Do not weigh every day. There will be some weeks when nothing happens and the scales appear to be stuck. This can affect your mood and produce that 'It's not working, so what's the point?' mind-set, which could precipitate a binge. You are allowing a mechanical object to measure and judge you.

A former client, Abby, says, 'I used to weigh myself twice a day. The scale was my emotional barometer. If I woke up feeling OK and the scales told me I had gained a pound, I'd experience a little sinking sensation in my stomach. If I planned to wear something I was saving for when I was slim and discovered I weighed more than I thought, I would take it off. It didn't matter how good I thought it looked on me before – once the scale delivered its verdict, I immediately began to think I looked fat.'

You will soon know when you have lost weight by the loose fit of your clothes and by other people's comments. Those scales can only tell you how many pounds you weigh. They do not tell you about the body's fat or muscle content so you don't know how much fat you have lost or how much muscle you have gained. You should only use your scales as an indication of your progress, not as a measure of your worth.

Get this: living slim is a *process*, not a result.

Eat Slowly

Everyone is so rushed today that eating becomes just one more quick fix, from the so-called 'nutritional' bar for breakfast, usually eaten on the way out the door, to the mad rush to the sandwich bar at lunchtime – with food brought back to the office to be consumed 'al desko' in five minutes flat.

Next time you are in a restaurant, look around you at how people eat. I know it's not very polite but it's fascinating to see how quickly people eat, particularly the fat ones. Their eyes are glued to the plate as the waiter serves them, and they use their forks as a shovel to transport the food into their mouths as quickly as possible.

It is really important to learn to relax when you are eating to allow your body to get the most from the food. When you sit calmly and eat slowly, your body can concentrate its blood supply on the stomach to digest the food properly. The digestive system consists of a collection of glands and muscles, which need a plentiful supply of oxygen – carried by the blood – and the appropriate hormones to enable it to work efficiently.

If you eat on the run or get up and rush around immediately after eating, oxygen is diverted from the stomach to the muscles required to move you around, such as your arms and legs, leaving the stomach bereft of the necessary oxygen to digest the food. This is what causes the indigestion, stomach cramps or acid reflux an hour later.

It is also important to sit up in your chair while eating rather than slouching on a sofa. Sitting upright allows gravity to help your stomach mix the food with digestive enzymes and pass this mixture along the intestine, where it is digested and absorbed.

Eating slowly will allow you to experience satiety – sensual satisfaction and fullness from eating – and avoid the bloated sensation so many people feel after eating on the run. The more you chew each mouthful and the more time you take over eating, the greater the feeling of fullness. The foods with the highest satiety values are those that stimulate more than one sense simultaneously – in other words, food that looks, smells and tastes good. If you like food with a 'crunch', it even sounds good. By sitting quietly and eating slowly, tasting every mouthful, you will get much more satisfaction from your meals.

It takes 20 minutes for the brain to register that there is food in the stomach and to switch off the hunger signals. The insulin released into your bloodstream when you eat filters slowly into the spinal fluid, and when it reaches a certain level this signals to the hypothalamus in the brain to switch off the hunger message. In those who are somewhat, shall we say, 'large-of-knicker', insulin enters the bloodstream more slowly and takes longer to filter into the spinal fluid. This is why fat people tend to eat more, and for longer, before feeling full.

The type of food you eat is also a significant factor. According to Dr Rosemary Stanton, an Australian food scientist, fast food like burgers and chips and sweet foods like chocolate bars are designed to need very little chewing, and dissolve rapidly in the mouth before being swallowed. This lack of mastication means the food has no time to release its odorous substances called 'volatiles' which are liberated when food is chewed thoroughly before being sent, via the nose, to the part of the brain that deals with satiety. Therefore you need to eat more of these kinds of foods before feeling satisfied that you have had enough.

Clients who are habitual bingers present me with the

biggest problem in getting them to slow down when eating. The binger mentality decrees that if you eat quickly, you can con your body into thinking that you are ingesting fewer calories. (Duh!) I tell them to slow down by deliberately chewing more slowly and not getting the next mouthful ready on the fork until they have swallowed the previous one and their mouth is empty. Or simply to put their fork in the other hand. You would be surprised how strange this feels. It concentrates the mind solely on what is happening. I also tell clients that, when eating in company, they should play a private little game and try to be the last one to finish.

Losing weight starts in the mind.

What are You Thinking?

Everyone has an inner voice that runs through their mind continuously. This little voice comments on what you see, judges other people, makes decisions, voices opinions and occasionally, when you are trying to sleep, drives you nuts with its constant chatter.

Because this little voice is continuous and relentless, its power can be deceptive, and it can lead you to think you have no control over it. The thoughts in your head are thoughts you have put there. You own them. They may be influenced by outside sources but, ultimately, you are the one who dictates the tone of these mind thoughts. You don't respond to what is happening in your world; you respond to your *interpretation* of what is happening. You may make faulty initial assumptions and then, because you believe and trust yourself, you treat these assumptions as fact and react accordingly. Therefore the words you put into your head are crucial to whether you succeed or fail, whether it is in losing weight or any other aspect of your life.

The trouble is that if you have been telling yourself for years how weak-willed you are and how you can never stick to a diet, every time you fail this proves that what you think about yourself is true. Even though you embarked on some bizarre weight-loss plan that nobody would be able to stick to, you still consider yourself weak and powerless. Haven't you just 'proved' it?

Your thoughts are the sum of your past experience, judgements, observations and reactions. Once you know you can control your thoughts, you can make sure they are the 'right' thoughts. Negative thoughts produce negative results. If you think, 'I can't stick to a diet, I'll always be fat, however much I try, nothing works,' you will find yourself being propelled straight to the biscuit tin. In the same way, positive thoughts produce positive results: 'I do not have to be fat any more. From now on, I am going to put healthy food into my body, I am going to plan a regular exercise routine and live as though I am already slim.' Sounds good, doesn't it?

Your mind will follow any instruction you mentally feed into it. It works below the level of consciousness, so if you focus firmly on the slim shape you wish to acquire, your mind will strive to achieve it. It is when you get bogged down with thoughts of chocolate biscuits that things go awry and your subconscious mind obligingly sets up a craving for you.

Once you are aware of this you can refocus your thoughts on your original slim image, and your mind will cheerfully switch back again to help you achieve it. Your subconscious mind doesn't care what you look like. It is simply waiting for you to direct it. If you keep feeding in positive thoughts, you will start to feel more optimistic, you will choose the correct food, you will feel more energetic and things will start working for you.

For every thought, there is a physiological reaction. Just for a moment, picture very hard that you are cutting a lemon into quarters, picking up one quarter and biting into it. Go on – your teeth are biting into the yellow surface and the bitter juice is going into your mouth. If you can imagine this vividly enough, I'm sure all the saliva has evaporated from your mouth and your tongue has clamped itself to the roof of your mouth in anticipation of the sour taste.

Another example: you are walking home on a dark night and sense that someone is following you. The hairs on the back of your neck start to prickle, your skin goes cold and your breathing gets shallow. It takes a moment or two to get back to normal when you realize there is no-one there.

Your nervous system can't differentiate between a

real or a vividly imagined experience. That is why just looking in the mirror and registering real or imagined rolls of fat can trigger a bout of depression, justified or not.

It takes quite a bit of practice to recognize your negative thoughts about your weight and appearance, especially if you are a binger and constantly berate yourself for overeating. These thoughts are second nature to you and feel natural. You have always thought that dwelling on these negative thoughts will lead you to act and finally change your bad habits. But has it?

Change the process. The truth is that once a thought, problem, vexation or feeling materializes in your mind, it stays there. You can dwell on it, you can act on it, you can decide not to act on it, you can find an alternative way of expressing it or you can attempt to deny its existence. But when you try to deny that something exists, it reappears in a different shape – in the form of 'fat thoughts'. The negative thought is there – simply acknowledge it and overlay it with a positive thought. Tell yourself that you don't have to think like that any more. From now on you are moving forward and the future looks good. Plant these positive thoughts very firmly in your mind. If you do this long enough and hard enough, everything else will fall into place.

Positive Affirmations

🥕   **If you tell yourself it is easy, it becomes so.**   🥕

The way to do this is actually to tell your mind what you want with 'positive affirmations'. Even if you don't believe them at the time, your subconscious mind will absorb the message and work to your advantage. The best time to do this is when you are lying in bed first thing in the morning in that sleepy period between awareness and actually getting up. Have four or five phrases that you fix into your head and repeat each day. Here are some examples but you can make up your own that are relevant to you:

I feel great. I am strong and fit and healthy.
I am in control of my life.
I am calm and relaxed.
I will only eat healthy food today.
Whatever happens, I can deal with it calmly and intelligently.
I look forward to each new day because of all the good
     things that are going to happen.
I can achieve and succeed in whatever I set out to do.

Repeat these phrases – or similar ones of your own – each day, even if you feel anything but 'great' or 'calm'. As you can see, these are all positive thoughts. There is nothing listed that sounds remotely like 'I will not eat chocolate today'. That is a negative thought. It is much better to say 'I will only eat healthy food today'. Suggest things that you *will* do, rather than what you *won't* do. By putting these suggestions into your subconscious mind, you are programming yourself to succeed this time. Just do it — it only takes a moment.

Get the Picture

As well as programming your mind with positive mental affirmations, you also need visual ones. When you look in the mirror, do you only notice the fat round your hips or do you see the person? Everyone has a mental image of themselves that might not correspond to the reality. The skinniest of models will tell you that her thighs are fat.

If your heart sinks at your image in the mirror, maybe it's time to change what you choose to see. Just as the words you put into your mind can influence how you feel, so the pictures you visualize in your mind have the same effect. If you imagine yourself as fat and lumpy, that is how you will remain. If you see the same, you will be the same. You have to see yourself differently. We discussed this in Chapter 1: you have to have something you are moving *towards*, a picture in your mind's eye of how you want to be, how you want to look. You have to visualize success — in detail — in order to succeed. If you have any doubts, it won't work.

Top athletes use this simple rule as a positive training technique to 'program' themselves for success. A tennis player will 'see' himself hitting an ace; a golfer will visualize sinking a putt every time. They plant these images into their minds over and over again. This sends a message to the brain that affects both energy levels and motivation, so that when they actually come to play, their bodies will automatically mirror the pictures in their minds. It's called winning the mind game.

By imagining yourself as slim, healthy and vibrant, you will automatically straighten your shoulders, pull in your tummy and look 10 pounds slimmer immediately. Pretend you are a dancer – this is just an exercise, I am not suggesting you take up ballet – and imagine a slim, elegant person who moves gracefully and to whom people are instantly attracted. Get a very clear image in your mind of what you want to look like. See yourself in the clothes you want to wear and imagine how you would feel walking into a room wearing those clothes and drawing admiring glances from the assembled crowd.

These exercises will store these images in your mental 'database' and encourage your body to gradually comply.

Control

The only person you can control is yourself. You can't change the world and you can't control the people around you, but you can control the way you respond to the world and everyone in it. 'I get so frustrated when my mother-in-law comes round. She always makes me eat.' No she doesn't. It is your response to your mother-in-law that causes you to eat. She doesn't tie you down and force-feed you. You do not have to react to anything or anyone by eating food you have chosen not to eat. Decide not to hand over your control-power to anyone else.

Program your mind that giving up sugar is free choice. Don't give in to the brainwashing – that if you don't allow yourself a certain food you will just crave it. You won't. You know you can eat it if you want to but you choose not to. It is much easier not to have any than to limit it. Having one bar of chocolate a day is as bad as eating it all the time. This will ensure you are still addicted to sugar, both in your body and in your mind. You might be able to stick to one bar for weeks at a time but when offered some cake at another time, you are compelled to accept it.

Limiting sugar never works because you have to exercise willpower and discipline every day for the rest of your life to stop yourself eating it at other times when you are tempted. If you don't have the willpower to stick to the previous diets you've tried then you've certainly not got enough to try and control a sugar craving. Stopping eating it altogether is much easier.

Get the myth of 'just one bite' out of your mind. There is no such thing as 'just a little taste'. If you like the taste you will want more, and if you don't like the taste you wouldn't have wanted to try it in the first place. A taste for sugar is an addiction that will last a lifetime unless you break it. While you still have that 'taste' in your brain, you won't get slim.

⊛ **Nobody eats just one peanut. Don't start.** ⊛

Banish the Brainwashing

1. You do not 'need' refined sugar for energy.
2. You will not be 'deprived' if you stop eating it.
3. It will not 'set up a craving' if you 'deny' yourself sugar.

If you believe these things, they will happen. Change your beliefs.

No-one deliberately wants to make themselves fat. Sometimes I say to a fat person, 'If you could turn back the clock to a time you were slim and I told you there was a way you could stay slim for the rest of your life, would you do it?' They always say 'Oh yes' and I reply, 'Well, there is. Just stop eating sugar.' That is all you have to do.

Experience a sense of power. It is a strong belief in your ability to succeed in everything you do – whether it is going for a new job, becoming slim or simply completing a task that has been bugging you – that will propel you to success.

See yourself as having the strength to resist all junk food and making wise food choices at every meal. Constantly reinforce the picture in your mind of this slim, healthy person. Feel that you *are* that person – not just the thought in your head. Feel that strength and feel that power. Induce a calm sense of commitment and inner strength that this is what you are moving towards. Let yourself dream – let yourself visualize – and know that it is your turn now.

Finally, be accountable. Know that if you don't stick to your regime, the consequences will be a steady increase in your weight. You will just get fatter and fatter, more tired, more depressed and possibly end up with cardiovascular problems or diabetes. The time to act is now.

Accepting your role in creating the shape of your body and acknowledging that you are accountable means that you get it. It means you understand that the solution lies within you. While others are still blaming stress, lack of willpower and diets that don't work for their inability to shift the pounds once and for all, you can slowly but surely move towards the slim corner you will inhabit for the rest of your life. In other words – *you get it.*

Telephone Conversation with Client

C: *I just can't stop eating chocolate. I'm so depressed. I'll never lose weight because once I start eating it, I literally cannot stop eating bar after bar until I feel sick. Then I vow never to touch it again, but the next day – off I go. What shall I do?*

Me: *So I presume you are now sitting there with the phone in one hand and a bar of chocolate in the other?*

C: *No, of course not, it's only 10 o'clock in the morning.*

Me: *So you can stop eating chocolate. Now all you have to do is find a way to stop eating it long enough to get slim.*

C: *Huh! If only it were that easy.*

Me: *It is. You simply decide that you don't eat chocolate any more. If that is the one food that is screwing up your shape, your health, your self-esteem and keeping you fat and miserable, then it isn't doing you any favours. If chocolate produced a life-threatening reaction in your body, you wouldn't think twice about avoiding it.*

C: *But it doesn't and I would feel deprived if I couldn't have my afternoon Twix – or two, or three.*

Me: *Fine, then stay fat. That's OK. It would be a very boring world if everyone looked the same. Enjoy your chocolate and resolve to be fat.*

C: *No – I hate being fat. Isn't there a middle way? Couldn't I just have chocolate once a day as a treat?*

Me: *You just said that once you start eating chocolate you can't stop. Elimination is always better than moderation* *if there is something you can't control. Someone giving up smoking doesn't allow herself one cigarette a day as a treat.*

C: *Are you saying I can never have chocolate again – ever – for the rest of my life?*

Me: *No. I am suggesting that you choose not to eat any chocolate today. You can only live one day at a time. When tomorrow comes, you will decide what you are going to do then, whether to have another choc-free day or go back to eating it. It's your choice. There's lots of other food you can eat which won't make you fat.*

C: *You're being very hard.*

Me: *Not at all. You have to decide what's important. Either you eat chocolate and stay fat or stop eating it and get slim. You can't do both. You've tried – it doesn't work. It's simply a matter of deciding which is more important to you: being slim, attractive and feeling good about yourself – or being fat, lumpy and miserable. It's your choice every time. No-one else cares what you look like.*

C: *You know what? You're a nasty cow!*

Me: *Absolutely!*

Chapter Six

Exercise – No Sweat, No Point

'And it came to pass, from the land of Adipose, the voice of the mighty prophet Gluteus Maximus: "Hear my words all ye potatoes-of-the-couch. Arise off thine lardy-butts and clothe thine limbs in garments of the finest Lycra. Then go forth and alight upon thine treadmills – for the Day of Marathon draws nigh."'

Get this: exercise is your secret weapon for losing weight and keeping it off. Every single person, without exception, who has lost weight and stabilized at the lower weight has found a way of incorporating some form of regular exercise into his or her lifestyle. Whether it is playing tennis, going to the gym or taking exercise classes, this must become part of your life. If your attitude is 'I can't be bothered' then that's fine: stay fat and unfit.

But before you make this decision, look around you next time you find yourself at a gathering of people of different ages, maybe a family wedding or a charity function. Check out the 50 and 60-year-olds and see which of them – men and women – are slim, have good postures, move easily and fluidly and look much younger than their years. Those are the ones who make time for regular exercise.

Then notice the plumper women with their heads poking forward and their shoulders sloping in that unattractive 'dowager's hump' – sorry Camilla P.B, nothing personal – and how they have to heave themselves out of a chair. Look at the men with their enormous tummies preceding them and wonder how on earth they can find their – never mind. Then decide how *you* would like to look.

Get up and Do it

🍎 **Do not let two days go by without doing some** 🍎
kind of exercise.

The key is regular exercise. In my experience, people will make the effort when they feel slim but not when they feel fat – regardless of the number on the scales at that particular moment. If you are serious about living slim then you need to acknowledge your excuses in this area. Yes, you have got time. I don't care about your bad back. So you sweat and your hair goes frizzy – so what?

Have You Got Time *Not* to Exercise?

If *your* excuse is that you haven't got time to exercise, what exactly are you saying here? Will you have time in the future to deal with the growing list of medical conditions that exercise is known to prevent? Can you take the time to recover from your heart bypass operation or the pain associated with your stiff back, hips or knees? If you don't exercise you are making a decision to compromise the quality of your life now and in the future. So don't say you haven't got time. You just haven't made the time – yet.

Fact: if you want to lose the fat on your body, you have to make the necessary changes to shift your metabolism into fat-burning mode. Very-low-calorie diets, missing meals, leaving long gaps between meals, detox regimes, foods containing refined sugar – all encourage your body to store fat. The only way to reverse this is to eat healthy food at regular intervals during the day and incorporate some sort of physical activity into your life. 'Bor-r-r-ing!!' No – it doesn't have to be. It is a matter of deciding what is important to you and what you are prepared to do to achieve it.

Find some sort of activity that you can do (and might even *enjoy*) on a regular basis and *make the commitment to do it*. If you intend to exercise during the day, schedule it in your diary. Once it is written down you won't be tempted to make other appointments at that time, so giving yourself a convenient excuse not to do it. Everyone – no matter how busy their schedule might be – can find three half-hour chunks of time during the week, *if they want to*.

Why Exercise Works

☾ **While you are exercising, you are not eating.** ☾

Exercise works on so many levels that it's worth understanding why I suggest you make that commitment to yourself. Right now, your body is probably not working at peak fat-burning efficiency – just a guess, of course! You could well have perfected the art of fat-*storing* though. The key to turning this around is to raise your metabolic rate.

Everyone has a 'basal metabolic rate'. This is the measure of how many calories your body needs in order to maintain its vital functions when you are doing nothing. Efficiency is based on how much muscle you have in your body – that is, skeletal muscle in your arms and legs, not organ muscle like your heart and intestines. Muscles contain special components called mitochondria, which are responsible for converting calories to heat and water. This is why you get hot and sweaty when you exercise –which makes it worth doing!

Working your muscles against some form of resistance causes more amino acids to collect in the muscle cells, making them denser rather than larger. Denser muscles contain more mitochondria so they burn up more calories. Therefore the more muscle you have, the more you can eat without gaining weight. Fat uses very few calories, so the more fat you have the slower your metabolic rate will be. Clearly, then, it is in your best interests to lose the fat and gain more muscle.

Strength, Suppleness and Stamina

There are three different ways to be fit – the three S's: Strength, Suppleness and Stamina. You really need a bit of each for optimum fitness.

Strength

You acquire strength by increasing your muscle power through working with weights, or against resistance by using the machines in the gym. You will need a trainer to guide you round the first few times until you are familiar with the different muscle groups and know what you are doing.

No, you will not develop bulging muscles from basic resistance training. To get an idea of how it works, imagine going to the supermarket and loading up with enough groceries to last you a month and carrying the heavy bags or boxes from your car into your house. You are using your arm muscles to do this and the heavy boxes act as resistance for your muscles to work against. If you carried several boxes in every day for about 20 minutes at a time, your arms would become pretty strong, though not bulgy.

Look at manual workers on a building site. They are immensely strong and can hold up a heavy hod full of bricks for long periods of time – it's a shame they can't do the same for their trousers. However, they are not in the same league as the body builders you see competing in contests, covered in Mazola. The more toned your muscles, the more shapely you will look – as opposed to flabby – but working on the machines to the exclusion of all other exercise will not get rid of fat.

Suppleness

Suppleness – being able to reach for the biscuit tin without putting your back out – will not burn fat on its own. However, it is an essential part of general fitness. Most people who spend a lot of their day in front of a computer screen or behind a steering wheel are notoriously stiff, leaving them prone to injuries. Your body was made to move, so some bending and stretching is vitally important to keep your joints flexible and your muscles long and lean. Yoga, Pilates, t'ai chi and jazz dance all achieve this and are useful for giving you a 'body awareness' that will help to keep you on track food-wise. After a lovely stretchy session you are unlikely to come home and dive into a plate of fried fish and chips.

Stamina

The *only* type of exercise that burns up the fat and increases your stamina is aerobic exercise, which is fast walking or jogging, cycling or rowing. Swimming is also classed as aerobic exercise but I am not keen on swimming as it combines too many irritating factors: you have to get wet, you won't do it for long enough and your body is reluctant to give up the fat when it is in cold water as it needs it for insulation. Then you have to dry your hair, and coming out of a cold, wet swimming pool into cold, wet weather is not the best incentive. Also, most people swim holding their bodies in the wrong position (trying not to get their hair wet?) and end up with neck pain or backaches.

Aerobic means 'with oxygen'. Fat burns in the presence of oxygen. Continuous body movement makes you breathe harder so more oxygen enters your bloodstream. This engages your muscles to use a stored carbohydrate called glycogen as energy. Once all the glycogen is used up, your body looks for another source of energy. It can't break down your muscle tissue because you are using it right now, so it turns to the fat. As explained earlier, your fat cells are designed to store fat and release it when it is needed for energy. Once your lipolytic (fat-burning) enzymes have been stimulated enough by the exercise to grudgingly release a little bit of fat into your bloodstream, this gets shunted towards your muscles. There it is grabbed by the mitochondria in the muscle cells and burned up as heat and energy.

Hence, the more muscle you have, the more fat you will burn. Exercise increases the amount of muscle, which in turn increases the efficiency of the fat-burning mitochondria in the muscle cells. This also makes your heart stronger while increasing the efficiency and capacity of your lungs. Still with me, everyone? Hang in.

The Feel-good Factor

A little more on the biology lesson: it has also been well

documented that exercise can lift depression and make you feel better about yourself because of chemical hormones called endorphins which are released into the bloodstream. Endorphins act on the brain rather like morphine, which explains why you don't feel any aches and pains while you are actually doing the exercise – it's the following day when you may feel a bit stiff and achy.

However, for all that to happen, you must be doing *continuous* – not vigorous – movement. People who don't exercise assume that aerobic exercise is frantic movement that you do until you collapse. It's just the opposite, in fact. Vigorous exercise such as tennis, football and squash is known as 'anaerobic' (without oxygen). Although it tones the muscles and stimulates the metabolism, it doesn't produce the steady and continuous increase in the heart rate and breathing rate, so it won't burn fat in the same way.

The minute you get out of breath, you are no longer burning fat – you have gone beyond what is alarmingly known as your 'cardio-endurance' level. This simply means that if you are puffing and panting and red in the face, you are 'without oxygen' and should slow down a bit to 'catch your breath'. Therefore, to burn fat, the exercise you do shouldn't be too fast or too slow, but moderate and continuous.

How Much Exercise do I Need?

You need a minimum of 30 minutes of aerobic exercise each time for your workout to be effective. It takes that long for your heart rate to gradually increase and stabilize at the higher rate for the duration of the exercise until you cool down. This is what increases your metabolic rate to burn up the food you eat rather than storing it as fat.

The key to using aerobic exercise to change how your body works is not, therefore, the number of calories you burn up *during* the exercise – although this is obviously a contributory factor. When you rev up your metabolism, it *stays* in that raised state for several hours after you have put your trainers away and got on with your life. So the pro-gressive benefit can add up to a loss of several pounds a year beyond that produced by the activity itself.

Some 'experts' suggest that this 30-minute stint can be broken down into three 10-minute sessions during the day. I do not see the logic in this – but then, I live in the real world. Picture it. There you are in your office at 10.45 hav-ing answered your letters and e-mails and ready for your 11 o'clock meeting. 'Aha,' you think, 'I have just got time to do a 10-minute aerobic session and get all hot and sweaty before my meeting!' As if! You need 30 continuous minutes to achieve the necessary physiological effect that will keep your metabolism chugging away for the rest of the day.

You will also read lots of advice in magazines or from the Ministry of Health that somehow exercise has to be within everyone's lifestyle with the minimum of effort. They advise you to take the stairs instead of the lift (why?), walk to the next bus stop (at least two minutes!), weed the garden (backache isn't a sign of fitness) or clench your bottom 10 times every hour (oh, please!). None of this will do anything to shift fat. For this to happen you need a concentrated, regular programme of exercise.

You need to focus on exercise that uses the large groups of muscles with minimal strain on any ligaments, bones and joints. The more muscles that are used, the greater the number of calories burned; the lower the perceived exertion, the longer and harder you can keep going. The best fat-burning exercise allows you either to burn a lot of calories in a short time, or to ensure that the movements are easy enough on the body to keep burning calories over a longer period.

What Type of Exercise Should I do?

✍ If you want to lose it, you have to use it. ✍

Not all types of exercise will help you burn fat. Let's look at some options in more detail.

Swimming: The major muscles in the lower body get very little workout, especially during the crawl. Moreover, you can't reach aerobic capacity using only the upper body – this might be the case for a very fit swimmer who does a mile in half an hour, but at a slower pace nothing is happening fat-wise.

Walking: Good, but it should be fast power-walking to be effective. A stroll before dinner won't work, except to delay your dinner.

Exercise bike: Only the muscles in the lower body are used.

Spinning: This is a class led by an instructor with everyone perched on stationary bikes. It is better than just sitting and pedalling on the stationary bike because you occasionally stand on the pedals to climb imaginary steep hills, and change hand positions. This is quite an intense cardio workout so take it easy to start with, and make sure the instructor knows you are a beginner – you won't be able to keep up with the advanced spinners the first few times.

Cross-country skiing: This burns a greater number of calories per hour than any other sport. There is a 'cross-country skier' machine in every gym.

Stairmaster: This provides complete flexion and extension of leg muscles but get advice from the gym or trainer because it's easy to do this incorrectly. It is unlikely that you would do this fast enough to burn significant amounts of fat.

Rowing machines: Great for burning fat as this movement engages most of the major muscle groups.

Roller-blading: Your legs go through the complete range of movement together with arm motion and upper body activity, which brings all the major muscles into play.

Treadmill: Instead of running, it is better to increase the elevation and 'power hike'. The treadmill inflicts the least pain at the highest intensity and burns more calories than the stationary bike. Some of the other machines cause more pain at lower levels, which limits their effectiveness.

Aerobics Classes

If you are a member of a health club, try an aerobic, body conditioning or step class. These are excellent for raising the metabolism and burning off significant amounts of fat, as is kick-boxing. A gentle workout on the machines in the gym for a few minutes before doing aerobic activity will get your muscles nice and warm. Make sure you have a good stretch after the workout because the key to maintaining a low weight and increased fitness is to develop long, *lean* muscles. 'Toned' means denser, not bulging, as we've said before.

When you consider the volume of fat to muscle, a compact little muscle weighing one pound would obviously weigh the same as one pound of fat – but that one pound of fat would take up five times as much space in your body. So you decide which substance you would prefer to create the shape of your upper arm.

Don't be intimidated by walking into a body-conditioning class seemingly full of toned, tanned triathletes with bare tummies like ironing boards. They go every day. You live in the real world. Introduce yourself to the teacher – she's the one with the microphone wrapped round her head – and tell her you're a new girl. Hopefully she will keep an eye on you and break down the moves so you get the hang of it.

It will take about four visits before it gels. Every sport has its own language; think of a volley and a lob in tennis, or a chip and a putt in golf. You will soon become familiar with a grapevine and a leg-curl. Do persevere

because the benefits far outweigh the initial awkward-
ness. It's even worth putting up with the dreadful music
(showing my age here – bring back Motown!).

Effective Exercise

Most people who join a gym at the beginning of January
drop out by the end of March because they can see no difference in themselves. They want to lose weight, tone up
and feel fitter but their exercise regimes fail to deliver. This
is not because they haven't stuck to the routine, but
because most of them do not push themselves hard
enough. To be effective, exercise must challenge the body
beyond what it is used to, and body shape will not
change without frequency and effort.

To lose weight and undo years of neglect you do have
to make an effort. Those new to exercise are usually
much fitter than they think they are, but have been so
used to hearing the cautionary 'Don't overdo it at first'
that they don't overdo it at all! The key for you is to get
the balance right.

According to Gina Kolata, author of *Ultimate Fitness:
The Quest for Truth about Exercise*, there is a lot of mislead-
ing marketing about what can be achieved with exercise,
and people's expectations have become inflated as a result.
Take the commonly held view that fat can be turned into
muscle. As Kolata says, 'You always see women on the
Stairmaster doing 40 or 50 reps and thinking that this is

going to "spot reduce" their thighs. In reality, there is a layer of fat covering the muscle tissue: cardiovascular work will burn off fat, while for muscle definition you need to do some "serious weights". These women working very slowly on this equipment are not building muscle, they're certainly not doing cardiovascular work, and if their aim is to thin down their thighs, they're going about it the wrong way. The truth is that if you are not sweating, you're not even burning the calories.'

To lose it, you have got to use it – hard! If you are unused to physical exertion you may feel quite tired after the first couple of sessions. This has more to do with the mind dealing with unfamiliar sensations than your working at your maximum capability. Obviously, you wouldn't ignore a sharp, localized and persistent pain which could indicate that some part of your body may be prone to injury, but aching muscles merely mean that the body is doing something it is not used to, and they will adapt if the exercise is repeated often enough. So go back and try again!

It is important to work to the point where you do feel reasonably exhausted. If you just hop onto a treadmill and amble along at a steady pace without really challenging yourself week after week, you will get little benefit. The best way is to imagine a scale of 0–10 where 0 is lying down and 10 is pushing it so hard that it's impossible to continue. Aim to work at a level somewhere between 5 and 7 so that it should feel 'reasonably difficult'.

The time that you spend exercising and the speed or intensity should increase in graduated steps as soon as the workout is easily achieved. You *need* to get hot and sweaty to get results, but don't set yourself impossible targets to the extent that you give up.

I think health clubs could do more in this area. In many cases, once they persuade you to part with your hard-earned dosh and hand you over to an instructor for an induction session, they seem to abandon you to get on with it on your own. If you want results, you should be shown how to achieve them, so don't be afraid to get one of the trainers to check your progress every now and again.

Matt Roberts, a personal trainer who has a chain of gyms, agrees that there is a problem in the industry but puts the blame more on inexperienced and unqualified trainers and indifferent management. 'The industry is unregulated,' he says. 'Many personal trainers have little or no experience and no qualifications. The fitness clubs *are* worried about the safety of clients but are not bothered about whether people are doing exercises correctly.'

Personally, I have been teaching exercise for many years and have also attended classes with instructors of all nationalities. In the 1970s and 80s, the American instructors were far superior to any others, but the proliferation of health clubs over the years has meant that managers don't always check whether the qualifications on a CV are necessarily accurate. I have experienced some pretty dire classes in swish New York clubs.

In my opinion, the best teachers are Australian as they have to renew their qualifications every year to make sure they are up to scratch. I have never had a bad

Australian instructor – so check out the accents in *your* local health club!

Having said all that, do bear in mind that fitness instructors do little else but train people to be fit. Fitness is their life and they assume you wish to become as fit and knowledgeable as they are. Don't let this put you off. They will discuss your muscle/fat ratio and talk about maximum heart rates, abs, pecs, lats and reps. You do not have to buy into this total exercise lifestyle – you just need to be fit *enough*. Even moderate exercise helps by shifting dietary fat and carbs away from the fat cells and into the muscles. You want to be free of disease, strong, supple and have loads of energy. Exercise is necessary for all of these but it doesn't have to take over your life.

What Happens if I Stop Exercising?

When I talk to people about getting fit, they often express a concern about what happens if they stop exercising. They fear that, once they start, they will have to keep going all the time or their bodies will instantly collapse into a mound of flab.

This is not so. Muscle and fat are very different substances and one can't turn into the other. When sportsmen stop training – and become television commentators – their muscles simply grow smaller again. As television commentators, they probably continue eating (and drinking) the same amount as they did when they were in full training and had lots of muscle to use up all the calories. Now they are not burning it up as they used to, they get podgy and flabby. All that is needed is a regular session you can slot into your life three times a week. This will be sufficient to keep your muscles toned and your body functioning in fat-burning mode.

Consistency is much more important than the type of exercise you do, and you must enjoy doing it or you will find every excuse to avoid it and eventually give up. Any form of exercise undertaken solely as a means of weight loss will not work because that is part of the dieting mind-set: 'Once I am slim I can stop doing this!'

These Shoes Were Made for Walking

I know that for some people the idea of joining a gym and competing with all those testosterone-fuelled egos is more than they could stomach, so may I stress that you do have other options. For all those who 'haven't got time to exercise' here is the solution.

If you are very pushed for time, factor the 'Jok' into your life as follows: Map out a route from your home round a 'block' of streets which covers about a mile – measure it roughly in a car. This is to be your regular 'beat' which you are going to cover at least five times a week. It will only take 15–20 minutes. The best time to do this is first thing in the morning before your brain can register any objection. From February onwards it gets light very early in the morning. Set your alarm clock for half an hour earlier, lay out your trackie-bottoms and trainers at the end of your bed, get dressed and go. Walk fast enough so your legs ache a bit. This is not just 'going for a walk'; this is your exercise time specifically to increase your stamina and burn up the fat.

Next, when this has become a daily habit, think of 'moving up a gear' to go a bit faster as you stride along. I don't mean run, just move slightly faster, employing a heel-toe movement – something between a jog and a walk, a 'jok'. Start by doing this from one lamp-post to the next, then go back to your walk. Try it again a bit further on, covering the distance between two lamp-posts. Over a period of time, try and build up so that you 'jok around the block', staying at the increased pace until you are nearly home, then slowing down a bit for the last few yards. You should be a bit puffy by then. This should only take 15–18 minutes. That's not much out of your day, is it? You will like the result – especially the shape of your legs.

I promise you, if you do it every day – or every other day – even just this few minutes round the block will make the greatest difference to the speed at which that weight drops off. The most difficult part is the motivation to propel yourself out of bed and towards the front door. Once you manage that, your legs will just carry you along. If you can bear to, arrange your face into a smile. This is very important (*see Chapter 5*): when your brain registers happiness, you smile. Therefore, when you smile, your brain assumes you are happy and will lift your spirits.

Don't try and go further than your designated 'block' because that might put you off doing it in the future – you 'haven't got time'. One mile – 15–18 minutes – is just do-able. If you prefer, go in the evening. That's fine, but make the commitment and *do it*. Ready? '1 2 3 o'clock, 4 o'clock jok, we're gonna jok around the block tonight. Get your tracksuit on – and join me Hon.'

When returning from your jok, walk around for a bit to allow your breathing to return to normal. Remember, it is moderate exercise that burns fat. If you are going so fast – running – that you get out of breath and are puffing like mad, it's not working. On the other hand, you should be slightly sweaty. The pace should be fast but steady. You will know when you are doing it right when your inner thighs don't rub together any more.

If you can get to the gym instead, then do 20 minutes on the treadmill, aiming to take it up to level 5–6 for at least 10 minutes before slowing down, then 10 minutes on the rowing machine, a quick stretch, then home.

There, it's done. A quick shower and you can get on with your day.

Take a 'Step' towards Fitness

As an alternative to the outside activity of a jog or walk, try a 'step' class or buy yourself a step to use at home. If you haven't seen a step at your local gym, it is a sturdy plastic-based platform with a non-slip covering and can be set higher or lower according to your level of fitness. In my opinion, a 40-minute step routine is *the* most effective, safest fat-buster of all. When you step up and down you use the largest set of muscles in your body – those situated in your legs and bottom. Working those muscles draws fat from all over the body to use as energy. Be warned though – you will sweat buckets. You can buy a step at any store selling sports equipment and there are lots of instruction videos on the market.

For me, as I am generally pressed for time, my step is the most used piece of equipment in my house. Just the knowledge that I can slip downstairs in the morning and pop a video into the machine with no-one watching as I prance around in my nightie makes life a lot easier than having to arrive at a health club at a specific time. After 40 minutes in the (video) company of a (preferably) American instructor, I have a shower and am ready to start my day.

Other Facts about Exercise
Healthy Bones

Weight-bearing activity such as walking, jogging, skipping or stepping is the only type of exercise that will increase your bone mass, which is vitally important in preventing osteoporosis. The constant tugging of the tendons against the bone encourages more minerals to enter the bone and, in turn, strengthens the weight-bearing joints in your hips and knees. With a stationary bike, the saddle takes your weight so you lose some of the benefit. The same applies to swimming as you are suspended in the water. Whatever type of exercise you choose, it must be done on a regular basis to bring about the necessary build-up in bone mass.

Weekly Full Workout

Whether you choose a step routine or a jok-around-the-block, you should also plan at least once a week to do a full hour of exercise, incorporating warm-up, aerobic activity, upper-body work using your arms, abdominal work on the floor and a final stretch and cool down.

You *need* to work on your abdominal muscles to keep your tummy flat. These should incorporate specific exercises that target the 'core' muscles, which will also strengthen your back. Nigella Lawson may be proud of her 'sticky-out tummy' but, believe me, this is not a shape you want to aspire to. Also, if your bottom tends to travel south for the winter, you need squats and leg-lifts to firm and tone your gluteal muscles so you look good in trousers.

The Time Frame for Success

Don't expect miracles overnight. You may not see any change in your body shape immediately. Just as when you start a new eating regime, your body has to adapt slowly to the increased activity, and may be suspicious at first. In the same way as you have to get past the 'plateau' before your weight starts to go down at a steady rate, so you have to encounter the exercise 'barrier' before your muscles start firming up. It could take about 12 weeks before you see a definite change in your shape.

The first three weeks of sticking to any new routine are the most difficult. If you're going to give up, it's likely to be during this period! You may decide you are too busy, too tired after a heavy day at work or simply that you don't feel very well. You certainly won't feel like going out after a binge, which will leave you heavy and lethargic and probably in your 'Sod it, who cares?' frame of mind. Be aware of these feelings and try to overcome them. Tell yourself to get your shoes on and get out that door, however ropey you feel. Once you start striding along, your legs will take over and you will feel better.

Set realistic targets and don't let your all-or-nothing perfectionist nature prevent you from lowering your goals if necessary. If you don't feel particularly energetic one day, just cover the route at a brisk walk instead of the walk/jog. This is not regressing – it's simply adapting your plan for how your body wants to operate on a particular day. You are human, after all, and it's better to modify your activity for that day than to miss it altogether, which is the easy way out – and *would* be regressing. Just go. You will be pleased you did.

Program your body for success. Resolve not to let two days go by without doing some kind of exercise. You will be surprised and delighted at the result.

Case Study

Loretta Weitzman, aged 55, mother of two grown children and three grandchildren.

'I am proud of the fact that I have reached the ripe old age of 55 without ever doing any exercise! I am not so proud that at 55 my waist measurement now exceeds my hips. According to my doctor, this fat round my middle is the "dangerous'" variety and I have to lose it – but I remember this doctor as a little schnip playing in his father's surgery – what does he know?!

'My family insist I change my eating and lifestyle habits. They say they want me around a bit longer – God knows why, they never pick up the phone! So all right, I'll do some exercise. I went with my daughter to her gym but the room was like some medieval torture chamber so I told her I'd meet her in the coffee area later. Honestly, there were about 30 of those treadmill things with some-one-in-Lycra pounding away on every one! What sort of mentality makes someone pay thousands of pounds a year to walk for miles without getting anywhere? Crazy.

'So what shall I do? I'll walk. I bought some clumpy trainer shoes. Do you know they are really comfortable? I was told I had to walk fast – "powder walking" or some-thing – so I walk fast. By the time I get to the pillar box at the end of my road I'm exhausted and my heart is thumping. I look around for a taxi to take me home.

Unlucky. I limp home and collapse into a chair. I wouldn't want you to think I'm unfit or anything!

'Having spent all that money on the shoes, I go again the next day, but now I'm smarter: I walk more slowly so I can get a bit further. No problem. When do the entries for the next marathon have to be in by? Sign me up!

'After two weeks I am walking round the block – quite fast. After four weeks, to my surprise, I could keep going for 45 minutes without getting breathless. I am also 12 pounds lighter and I can actually fit into that beige suit I haven't worn since Anthony's Bar Mitzvah – you know the one, with the braid round the lapels?

'Don't laugh, I went to an exercise class – but the trouble is, I don't speak Aerobic. The teacher called out "grapefruit" and "ham-curl" and "heel-dig" – I had no idea what she was talking about so I just marched – to my car. I'll stick with the walking.

'It is now six weeks and I can jog from my house to the Post Office and back. That is a mile and a half and did you notice I said jog?! Can you believe that? The first time I tried to jog I thought I was being followed – but it was just my bottom jiggling. I do it three times a week and I have lost 16 pounds! I can't tell you how much better I feel. I don't get puffy anymore and my legs are so much firmer. I am definitely going to continue with this. Why didn't someone tell me about the benefits of exercise earlier? Oh, you did?'

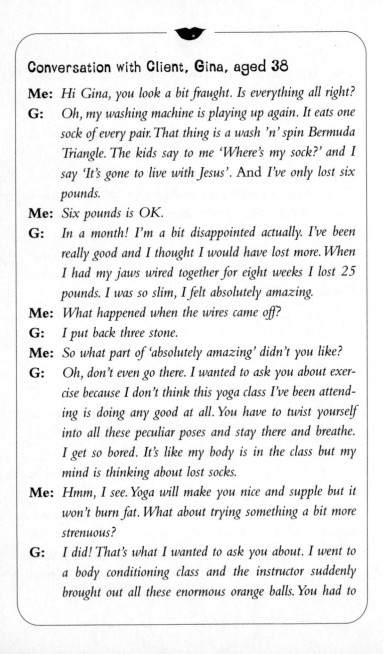

Conversation with Client, Gina, aged 38

Me: *Hi Gina, you look a bit fraught. Is everything all right?*

G: *Oh, my washing machine is playing up again. It eats one sock of every pair. That thing is a wash 'n' spin Bermuda Triangle. The kids say to me 'Where's my sock?' and I say 'It's gone to live with Jesus'. And I've only lost six pounds.*

Me: *Six pounds is OK.*

G: *In a month! I'm a bit disappointed actually. I've been really good and I thought I would have lost more. When I had my jaws wired together for eight weeks I lost 25 pounds. I was so slim, I felt absolutely amazing.*

Me: *What happened when the wires came off?*

G: *I put back three stone.*

Me: *So what part of 'absolutely amazing' didn't you like?*

G: *Oh, don't even go there. I wanted to ask you about exercise because I don't think this yoga class I've been attending is doing any good at all. You have to twist yourself into all these peculiar poses and stay there and breathe. I get so bored. It's like my body is in the class but my mind is thinking about lost socks.*

Me: *Hmm, I see. Yoga will make you nice and supple but it won't burn fat. What about trying something a bit more strenuous?*

G: *I did! That's what I wanted to ask you about. I went to a body conditioning class and the instructor suddenly brought out all these enormous orange balls. You had to* *perch on one and roll around, which I thought was completely pointless. Then you had to drape yourself over the ball and do abdominal crunches. Obviously I fell off, and now I've really hurt my back. A bloody great ball is hardly a stable piece of gym equipment, is it?*

Me: *Did the teacher know you were a beginner?*

G: *She didn't ask. I'm fed up with exercise.*

Me: *Well, you'd better see a physio about your back, and once you're better why not try something a bit more fun, like a jazz dance class?*

G: *I could do I suppose, but I think if God had meant us to stretch our arms up, He would have arranged for chocolate to grow on trees!*

Chapter Seven

You Don't Take Orders from a Biscuit

Well, you know what they say: the reason married women tend to weigh more than single women is because single women come home, see what's in the fridge and go to bed – whereas married women come home, see what's in the bed and go to the fridge…

Wouldn't life be easy if you alone determined what food you kept in the house and what you ate? If you didn't have any other factors involved such as having to shop and cook for your family, go out with friends, deal with working lunches? Then you could buy only healthy, non-fattening food and not find notes left in the kitchen saying, 'Mum, don't forget Emma and Sasha are coming for tea. Can we have pizza and Ben & Jerry's Chunky Monkey ice cream please.'

Well, life isn't like that – and how boring it would be if it were. Everybody faces daily challenges and you shouldn't underestimate how difficult it is to stick to a healthy eating plan when everyone around you is tucking into melted cheese.

You should, however, try to avoid the 'all-or-nothing' mentality. Losing weight doesn't mean cutting out every food you enjoy – only those foods that do you harm,

whether it's mentally, by pulling you down, or physiologically, by encouraging your body to store fat. If cheese
isn't your binge food and you want a pizza now and
again, even though you consider it 'fattening', then go
ahead. It's not so much which food you eat or the number of calories it contains, it's the effect a particular food
has on you. If it prompts you to overeat, now is the time
to choose something else!

In a perfect world you would be able to eat whatever
you liked and not put on weight. This is not a perfect
world and there is no perfect diet. You only have a problem with food if you make food a problem. Deciding you
can eat whatever you like provided it doesn't contain sugar
will solve that problem, although you will need to stay
aware of portion sizes and fat content if you want to lose
weight.

As I explained in the 'Living Slim' eating plan (*see
Chapter 4*), the main source of energy for your muscles is
carbohydrates, which are broken down into their com-
ponent sugar molecules and transported into the bloodstream. Your pancreas reacts by producing insulin to
make sure your blood sugar levels don't get too high, and
this prompts the body to store any surplus sugar as fat.
Eating carbs like bagels or potatoes at every meal
because you think they are low in fat puts your body
into a constant state of fat storage. It also prompts a craving for more of the same type of food.

Being in Control

✾   **You don't need to eat to please anyone else.**   ✾

The most important point, therefore, is not so much what you eat as to be *in control* of what you eat. To do this you may have to learn to be more assertive around other people. Sometimes saying 'No thanks' to unwanted food can be much harder than resisting internal temptations. Sometimes you will need to behave differently from the people you are with in social situations. When you are eating with other people, you have the right to ask for what you want to eat, even if this conflicts with what others want or expect. You do not have to drink alcohol if you don't want to. You do not have to eat the usual tea-time fare at someone's house, even though they may have gone to a lot of trouble to prepare it. If you would be desperately embarrassed to sit there with an empty plate, then go for a bread option (sandwich or bridge roll) rather than a sugar option (cake).

Many of my clients are afraid to say what they want for fear of another person's disapproval. They think it is disrespectful not to eat food that is offered. However, it is neither right nor necessary to put the feelings of anyone else before your own good health. If you have decided not to drink alcohol or eat food containing sugar, then you can always say how lovely the item looks but that you are absolutely full right now.

This fear of offending people can often extend to strangers. One of my clients was too scared to send back some unordered chips in a restaurant in case the waiter got annoyed. You do not have to take responsibility for other people's needs and sensitivities. Your health and how you feel are more important than the approval, or disapproval, of anyone else.

Just Say 'No'

Saying 'No' can be the hardest aspect of changing your eating habits. It is worth practising how to refuse diplomatically. You will cope better if you plan in advance what you are going to do or say. If you want to say 'No' then say it with conviction. Wistful statements like, 'Well, I shouldn't really' or 'I'm not supposed to eat that' only invite people to try and persuade you that you should. If you do not want to eat something, make it clear by using 'No' in your answer. Give a reason if you want to, but don't use any words to soften your refusal that may end up with you having to say 'Yes' after all.

Compile a list in your mind of each area of potential conflict, such as dinner parties, business lunches, eating out with friends. The secret of success is behaving as you choose to behave and not just going along with everyone else's whims. Consider carefully whether anyone actually needs to know that you are trying to lose weight. Once you tell people you are on a diet, for some reason they tend to start advising you how to go about it! 'You shouldn't cut out all carbohydrates, you need them for energy,' someone will say when you refuse the bread roll.

Or you will hear comments like, 'I suppose you're not having any birthday cake.' 'Oh, you never eat anything!' (I get this from people I have met for the first time!)

Do not let yourself be influenced by such comments. It is up to you to choose what is appropriate to eat every time. If you are avoiding a particular food because, in your case, it starts you overeating, then you don't have to eat it, whatever anyone says.

Strategies for Success

You can't cure an ingrained bingeing habit – the same as you can't 'cure' an alcoholic or drug tendency. You can only 'manage' it by developing strategies that will help you stay in control. Let's look at some of the strategies you will need to see you through the difficult times when you could so easily allow yourself to be sucked back into your old behaviour.

Dealing with High-risk Times

Eating is a learned response. If you always have a choco-late biscuit mid-afternoon, your body will come to expect that and set up a craving. Past behaviour may pre-dict, but needn't determine, future behaviour. To change these habits you need to identify your own pattern of eating and have a plan to counteract these crave times. When are your high-risk times, those times when you

are most likely to eat fattening food? For most people
these are:

★ Late-night eating
★ Snacking while watching television
★ Studying
★ Alone and bored
★ Eating in restaurants
★ On the way home from work
★ When the kids are in bed
★ When it's dark and quiet and there is no more
    stress
★ When you are feeling empty, hungry, lonely,
    depressed, stressed and anxious, edgy and irritable
★ Fearing deprivation: 'What's the point of going
    out if I can't eat anything?'

Identify your personal high-risk times so you can plan
and work around them. If you've got into the habit of
eating while you watch television in the evening, plan a
low-fat snack in advance and have it ready for when you
start looking around for something to nibble on (before
those chocolate ads come on!). You will gradually look
forward to this and enjoy it, rather than struggling to resist
then giving in and stuffing your face the whole evening.

    Have an 'emergency' food ready for edgy times when
you arrive home with a parking ticket or when you walk
into a room and see a stain on the carpet with the
unmistakable odour of cat pee: any situation when you

experience a jangling of nerves and *need* to eat something to calm you. A slice of rice cheese between two thin rice cakes is better than diving into the biscuit tin.

Do not have high-risk foods in the house. Even though you may not think about them most of the time, you know that when that craving hits, you will be heading straight for the drawer where you stashed the chocolate-coated peanuts. If your trigger foods are in the house – those foods that start you off on an eating binge – then sooner or later you will go for them. Someone trying to give up smoking does not leave a packet of cigarettes on the kitchen windowsill. The food you surround yourself with is the food you will gravitate towards and overeat. If you had to go to a supermarket to get it you might think twice, and the binge could be averted.

'But I've got to have chocolate in the house for the children.' Why? So they will have to go through the same misery with their weight as you are doing? That makes sense!

Get this: if you want to lose weight, the first place you look is at your excuses.

Dealing with Stress

In a stressful situation, don't turn to food.
It is more stressful being fat.

Do you think only food can make you fat? Wrong. If you have a persistent little roll of fat just below your navel that refuses to budge no matter how many abdominal crunches you do, this could be caused by stress.

When you feel that tight, shaky feeling inside you as you race towards a deadline, an appointment or an impending argument, the stress-induced hormones adrenaline and cortisol pour into your bloodstream to prepare your body for the 'flight or fight' response. This in turn releases stored glycogen to raise blood sugar levels and to give your muscles an energy boost. This was fine for our ancestors, whose response to stress was physical action. As stress today is mainly mental or emotional, the body has to cope with this excess of blood sugar by releasing yet more insulin to take the glucose out of circulation and store it conveniently in your fat cells.

Elevated levels of the stress hormone cortisol increase the storage of fat in the stomach area. This is because fat cells located deep in the abdomen seem to have more receptors for cortisol than those at more superficial levels in the body. The same effect is created by stimulants such as caffeine and nicotine, which is why you may feel hungry after drinking coffee – and why teenage girls who take up smoking thinking it is going to keep them slim are sadly mistaken.

Clients have told me they lead stressful lives. I get that. Some amount of stress is inevitable. We all experience it, at different times, and a lot of the time it's not under our control – that's why we get stressed! But, most of the real stresses have been removed from everyday living. You don't have to kill an animal for supper tonight and I haven't seen anyone driving to work in a horse and cart recently.

Most of the stress we experience today is of our own making. We tend to confuse stress with responsibility. All adults have some responsibilities, such as work, mortgages and children, and your stress levels are dependent on how you handle these normal processes. Food, in this case, doesn't change anything – except to make you more stressed when you get fat. Your brain is wired to handle stress and it needn't involve chocolate. When you feel fit and strong, mentally and physically, you can handle anything. The very substance you use as a prop – sugar – will pull you down mentally and make you lethargic.

Stress takes many forms and is often exacerbated by the way you think and feel. Although you can't entirely eliminate stress, you can learn to manage it so it doesn't become an overwhelming or destructive force in your life. The way to do this is to analyse each situation and attempt to separate the true facts from any emotional interpretation you might put on it. Stop for a moment and ask yourself what is *really* happening here.

An example: your project plan was rejected by your boss, even though you had worked night and day on it for weeks and believed it was in line with what he wanted. You are now irritated and depressed and thinking, 'I can never get anything right.' Is that really the case or is that an irrational thought you have put into your head? Change it around by saying to yourself, 'The last one was very successful. I'll go and ask him where this one is wide of the mark – then I'll have another go at it.'

Try and disperse feelings of frustration and depression as soon as possible. The faster you can act to prevent yourself sinking deeper into misery and change to a more positive way of thinking, the sooner your stress level decreases – as will the likelihood of it ending in a binge.

Aim to set yourself up for a calm day in the first place, by programming your mind with the affirmations referred to in Chapter 5. Alternatively, you could practise the following deep-breathing technique, which actors use before going on stage:

Take a long, slow, deep breath, pushing your tummy out at the same time so the breath goes into the lowest part of your lungs first and fills up from there. Hold the breath for a moment then gently blow the air out through your mouth, at the same time pulling in your tummy. This is the opposite of how you usually breathe, which is just using the upper part of your lungs in your chest. Do this four or five times, sensing how your mind and body seem to relax as the tension flows out of you on the out-breath. You will then be able to think more clearly and deal calmly with whatever needs to be done.

Dealing with Cravings

♧ **Some food can go from fingers to thighs in** ♧ **30 seconds.**

Cravings start with your eyes. You see some delicious-looking fattening item and the thought forms in your brain, 'That is a delicious-looking fattening item I would like to eat.' Your memory then kicks in and reinforces how that particular item tasted when you last ate it, conveniently not recalling how it subsequently attached itself to your thighs causing untold anguish two days later. All you remember is the pleasant taste. As explained earlier, for every thought there is a physiological response: so your mouth starts watering, you get an empty, anticipatory feeling in your stomach and you actually feel a little bit weak with desire. And then the excuses begin in your mind as you try to rationalize why you should eat this food:

'I'm absolutely starving'

'I've been so good for three days'

'I'll just have one bite and throw the rest away' (Yeah, *right*!)

'If I have this now, I won't have dinner later'

'I can still get into my black trousers'

Do you give in? Usually. Do you have to? No.

A strong compulsion to eat is referred to as a craving, implying that we have no choice in the matter. The substance seems to control you and tell you that you simply have to eat it. Sometimes the craving can be so intense that you start shaking in the same way a drug addict behaves when deprived of a fix. It doesn't really matter whether certain foods do have this power over you because you are addicted to their chemical make-up, or whether you feel compelled to eat them for psychological reasons. The effect is the same: you lose all rational control and have to eat.

What you have to realize is that a craving is a *feeling*, not an order to be obeyed. It is a short period in your life, a moment in which you decide whether you will eat this item or not, a moment that will determine what you eat for the rest of the day, how you will feel about yourself afterwards and how you will look in the future. It can be an 'Oh sod it!' moment or an 'I don't eat that stuff' moment, depending on how you have programmed your mind.

Yes, it is possible to program your mind to resist cravings. It is absolutely crucial to grasp this point so that you see the situation is not hopeless. Things can be changed and you can choose whether you want them changed or not. Once you realize you have this choice, you will feel much more confident about your ability to alter your behaviour and get your food craving under control.

The other good news is that you don't have to be strong every single hour of every single day. You are not fighting cravings all the time, only at specific 'impulse moments'. These brief moments may happen two or three times a day at first but will gradually disappear once the sugar residue is out of your system.

A craving doesn't come out of the blue. You actively have to think 'I want to eat that' for the craving to begin. The thoughts in your mind are the thoughts you have put there. Knowing this, you can change them to different thoughts. It can be done. It means learning to recognize a crave-thought when it pops into your mind and immediately substituting a more positive thought, before the physiological effect takes place.

Don't Take the First Bite!

To be more specific, you should have a particular phrase that you repeat over and over again until it becomes automatic. Most of my clients opt for 'Don't take the first bite'. They know full well that it is the initial taste of sugar that starts them off on a raid-the-kitchen splurge. No-one can stop at just one chocolate raisin. If the initial taste doesn't take place, the binge doesn't happen. Practise saying 'Don't take the first bite' whenever you see anything containing sugar, whether in a shop window or in front of you at a tea party.

Put the thought very firmly in your mind that you don't eat that stuff. You know you can if you want to but you choose not to at this moment. You are not imposing a life sentence on yourself. You want to be slim and that is more important than a transitory taste of something sweet. So 'don't take the first bite'.

Make up your own phrase if you prefer. Young mums tend to tell themselves firmly, 'You are not a dustbin' when confronted with the remains of their child's tea. Decide on a phrase that is personal to you. It has to be a command. 'Stop now!' prevents some people putting whatever it is into their mouth. Others prefer 'Remember, you don't eat that stuff – move on!' Choose a phrase and repeat it over and over again every time you see some tempting food, whether you are passing a bakery shop, standing next to the confectionery at the supermarket checkout or simply watching someone at the next table tucking into your favourite dessert. After a while the phrase will automatically pop into your head – and save you a lot of grief.

Don't pick - ever. Think of your fingers as 'weapons of mass consumption'.

Visualization

Use visualization to reinforce the message. Shut your eyes and think back to the last time you grabbed some fattening item and stuck it into your mouth. Was it that one remaining slice of cake that it was 'a shame to waste' (and therefore became 'waist') or those few chips left on your child's plate? Then picture yourself saying very firmly 'Don't take the first bite', picking up the cake or chips and pushing the food down the waste disposal unit or deep into the bin. See, how painful was that? No problem. Repeat this scenario several times in your mind.

Change Your Inner Voice

Sometimes your thoughts simply need a different response: a contradiction of the original thought. You should make this immediate and definite. For example:

'Ooh, that looks yummy.' 'No it doesn't. It is just a lump of fat and I don't need it.'

'I'm on holiday. Surely I should be able to eat what I like.' 'Come on – I have done so well up to now, I am not going to undo everything I have achieved for a plate of chips and a few glasses of wine.'

'I ought to eat it – she went to all that trouble.' 'Why should I let someone else make me fat?'

'It's all paid for – it would be silly not to eat it.' 'Don't be ridiculous! That is "fat" thinking.'

If you make your inner voice strong and positive all the time, eventually a change will come over you and the new thought patterns will have become your reflex responses. Every time you resist a craving, it will be easier the next time.

Distractions

Another way of dealing with cravings is to distract yourself with some sort of activity. These are the ones that work:

★ Mental – get in front of the computer, send e-mails to all your friends or play computer games. ('Freecell' – a form of patience – is on most computers and every permutation can be done. I've never been beaten. How sad is that?! But it keeps me busy enough to forget the call of the fridge.) If you are not into computers, keep a book of crossword puzzles handy or a permanent jigsaw puzzle on your table. The jigsaw works for most people but the trouble is, if a neighbour pops round to borrow a cup of money, or whatever, she can still be found there six hours later muttering 'I'm sure this piece goes here' or 'I'll leave you to do the sky.'

★ Exercise – get out of the house, away from the food

and go for a power walk. Take your personal stereo
and a talking book from the library. This is your chance
to catch up on the latest bestsellers.

★ Distraction - phone someone - anyone. You can't
concentrate on two things at the same time and you
wouldn't do something as disgusting as eating while
talking on the phone. Would you? Or tidy your make-up
drawer. You are never going to wear that colour
lipstick, so chuck it out.

★ Laughter - a video that makes you laugh changes the
brain chemistry in the same way that the food would do.

★ Change the anticipated taste - for example, if you
crave chocolate, pop a pickled onion into your mouth
instead. Then see if you still fancy the chocolate!

The following are the ones that *don't* work – the advice
usually given in women's magazines to counter stress:

★ Have a warm, relaxing bubble bath. (It's the middle of
the day for God's sake!)

★ Get your partner to give you a soothing massage. (My
partner is at work. Will the dishwasher repair man do?)

★ Light some scented candles. (What on earth for?)

★ Think of a pleasant scene. (I am - it's me eating
cheesecake.)

★ Listen to classical music. (While I'm eating the cheesecake?)

Do what works. Deal with cravings as soon as they pop
into your head. Remember, it's one decisive moment

that can change your life for the better or make you feel worse. Get rid of the crave-food. Sweep it straight into the bin. Yes, it is a shame to waste food but it is better in the bin than on your hips. If this is not possible, remove yourself from the site of temptation – now. Do not make bargains with food – 'If I eat that now I won't eat anything later.' You are intelligent – food isn't.

Dealing with Tricky Situations
Eating Out

✵   **Eat before you go. If you arrive empty you**   ✵
will leave fat.

Before you go anywhere, have a snack. Yes, even before going to a restaurant. If you go straight from work having not eaten since lunchtime, you will dive into the breadbasket, smear butter on the contents and consume hundreds of calories without being aware of what you are doing. Even if you are going out from home, have a snack about an hour before you leave for the restaurant. This sounds strange as you are 'going out to eat', but I promise that if you arrive hungry, you will leave fat. You never know exactly when you will be eating. The table may be booked for 8 o'clock, but by the time everyone arrives, the menu is brought and choices are made, it could be another hour before the first course actually arrives.

If you have had a few ounces of cottage cheese or a yoghurt and half a banana at 7 o'clock, you will be quite comfortable waiting for the food to come without that ravenous feeling in your stomach, and it will not spoil your appetite for your meal.

If you have weight to lose, when you go out to eat it is a good idea to decide beforehand what you are going to have so you won't be influenced by other people's choices. You usually know what sort of restaurant you are going to, and most places serve protein of some sort. Decide on a starter of melon, smoked salmon, asparagus or just ask for a mixed salad. For a main course, fish, chicken, lamb or whatever – with lots of different vegetables. If you are unsure, then decide to make this a 'carb' night and order pasta with a big salad. Not many people go for dessert nowadays but if your friends do, opt for plain berries if available or fruit salad – or, nothing.

One of my clients swore she never had desserts, even though she ate out at least three times a week. Apparently, asking for a spoon and tasting everybody else's did not count in her eyes! 'It was only one little teaspoon!' And how many people were round the table on the last occasion? 'Er – ten.' Fine! You just don't get it, lady!

It is more difficult at dinner parties or catered functions where you have no choice, but if you stick to the same rules you can stay in control. Always eat before you go out, even if you are only visiting close friends. You know there will be snacks like crisps and nuts laid out temptingly in front of you, and you never know what time the food will actually be served. Make it a rule not to go anywhere hungry.

Obviously, you do not want to turn into one of those guests-from-hell who are on some weird detox or food-combining regime and make life difficult for any hostess, but just say 'No thanks' when offered something you don't want to eat, and smile sweetly at any jibes you might attract from the other not-so-slim guests who are stuffing their faces and simply want you to do the same. **You need never eat to please anyone else.** If you can say to your hostess 'No potatoes please' without her getting offended, then do. If not, just leave them on your plate. Asking for second helpings of vegetables will absolve you from not eating the fattening stuff later.

Any conversation that starts with 'I'm trying this new diet…' is extremely boring and prevents the other guests from relaxing with their food. If you are helping yourself from dishes on the table, pile your plate with veg or salad so no-one can remark that you are 'not eating anything'.

How will you deal with the delicious desserts your friend has made 'especially for you'? Simple. If they contain sugar, you don't eat them. You should feel free to eat whatever you like, and if that means not having dessert because there is no sugar-free alternative, then so be it. Embarrassing? No – it's more embarrassing being fat. Don't go into lengthy explanations. Just say that you are full up after the first two courses and although everything looks absolutely wonderful, you just couldn't eat another thing. Your favourite chocolate mints on the table in front of you? Pass them to the person next to you and make sure they end up at the other end of the table. Don't take the first bite.

If anyone questions your behaviour, you can always say you are being tested for an allergic reaction to sugar – which is true. When you eat it, you break out in fat.

Entertaining

In a way it is easier eating at restaurants or in other people's homes. Once you have declined the tempting offering, they just take it away and you can't go back and raid the fridge three hours later, as you might do in a moment of weakness in your own home.

When you entertain, don't serve your obvious favourites then try not to eat them. You won't succeed. There is plenty of food you can eat that is perfectly acceptable as dinner-party fare. If you feel obliged to make some creamy dessert, make sure you also prepare a large platter of fruit to leave on the table, so your guests can help themselves. Use colourful fruit such as pineapple, melon, mango, kiwi, tangerine segments, small bunches of green and black grapes, and any type of berry. Remove the skin where necessary and cut the fruit into chunks on the plate. Provide plenty of cocktail sticks and watch how people tuck in. Your women friends will be particularly appreciative, and you can nibble without causing too much damage. As soon as your guests have departed, put that creamy dessert either in the bin or in the freezer – not down your throat.

Holidays

Many of my clients find holidays difficult to cope with when it comes to their eating plans. Ah, holiday-time – the illusion that because you're in a different place, you'll be a different person. The reality is you normally revert to the person who eats without being aware. This can be tricky but only if you have the 'I should be able to enjoy myself and eat whatever I like' mind-set. Tell that to your body. You may be on holiday but your fat cells aren't.

When you arrive, find the nearest supermarket and buy some bottled water and fruit to keep in your room. Stick to your plan of eating healthy food and don't resort to eating junk just because someone else is. If your children have chips with every meal, you do not have to pick. What is your phrase? 'Don't take the first bite' or 'You are not a dustbin'. You can enjoy yourself without coming home 10 pounds heavier.

Clients have complained that eating in cafés, restaurants or hotel dining rooms twice a day with small children makes it practically impossible to stick to their eating blueprint while travelling. In that case, negotiate with your partner over childcare. If you look after the kids in the morning while he goes and plays tennis or whatever, he could take them off for lunch while you grab an hour's relaxation by the pool with some fruit and cottage cheese. In this way you avoid temptation and can read your book in peace for a while.

The important thing is to keep positive messages in your mind all the time. Your thoughts will determine what you do. If you think 'I'll eat whatever I like and go back on my diet when I get home', you will find this very hard to do. Eating is a habit. Even if you are only away for a week, your body can quickly get used to eating chips at lunchtime. That is what it will come to expect and it will set up a craving when you are back home.

Stick to healthy eating as far as possible, wherever you are. An extra glass or two of wine won't hurt but make wise food choices at every meal.

Dealing with Your Family
Couch-potato Husbands

When clients say to me, often in despair, 'Please will you do something with my husband?' I am never quite sure what they have in mind! Then the tirade begins, 'He comes home from work and just slumps in front of the telly with a zapper in each hand. He eats all the wrong things, he drinks too much, he never does any exercise and he really needs to lose a stone but when I try and tell him…' Blah, blah, blah.

Well, that's your first mistake, girl! You can't tell him. You can't tell anybody how to eat. A woman's place is in the wrong – believe it. In my experience, when men make the commitment to lose weight, they generally succeed by working it out for themselves. All you can do, if you are the main shopper in the family (even though you also work full-time, I know, I know), is to make sure there is healthy food in the fridge and freezer for him and your children to make their own choices.

Kids' Mealtimes

And talking about children, that is another minefield for mums. Yes, I know it's hard being a stay-at-home mum with small children. It *is* dispiriting to spend hours cooking nourishing meals for your baby to spit in your hair. It is extremely difficult not to become a walking swing-bin for Marmite soldiers, half a fish finger, bits of cheese stuck to crusts and a splodge of banana. Sometimes you forget what it's like to talk to someone who isn't dribbling. But this is what you chose to do.

So let's get one thing clear: if you ignore every strategy I offer in this book, please take note of this one. *Do not eat from your children's plates.* Get this: there is no point sitting with a healthy tuna salad in front of you, nicking chips from your son's plate then wondering why your weight isn't going because you 'only had a salad for lunch'.

Make some rules:

★ Sit down and have a quiet snack or a meal before feeding your children.

★ Pick up their plates and sweep all the leftovers into the bin without looking at them.

★ Regardless of when the children eat, make sure you stick to the rule of eating every three hours.

This applies equally to working mums who should make it a top priority to sit down quietly when they get home and have a prepared snack. Just that 10-minute respite will calm you down and complete the transition between work and home, so preventing that endless picking of food between homecoming and dinner. You will still have time to test the children on their six-times table, undo the knots in their trainers with your teeth and find 20 small things that can fit into a matchbox which should have been handed in yesterday.

I am not going to tell you what to give your children to eat. You know this. Anyway, most children prefer to eat products that they see other children sing about and throw into the air in television commercials. They refuse your delicious grilled fish, but will cheerfully eat a cheese sandwich if it has been stuffed down the side of an armchair for two weeks.

All I will advise on the subject of feeding your kids is this: don't use sweets as a bribe or reward – and don't withdraw them as a punishment. This will endow sugary foods with an emotional value that may carry over into adulthood – and look where that got you! Children learn what they live. They copy their parents and, unfor-tunately, many parents are unwittingly encouraging the same habits that led to their own weight problem. Every fat child I see has a fat parent – usually the mother. If you want them to be free, you have to provide the means of escape. Our grandparents didn't really know about nutrition. You do, so use that knowledge to help your kids make informed and healthy choices. You are the food buyer, not them. I have known homes that are junk-free and the children don't seem to be deprived or rebellious. They just assume all families eat the same way.

Learn from Your Children

A former client, Cassie, always took a chocolate treat for each of her three children when she collected them from school. The problem was, she usually took one for herself as well and sat in the car picking at chocolate buttons until the children came out. This did not do much for her waistline, but she always seemed to get the 'munchies' at around 3.30pm. I advised her that if she wanted to continue poisoning her children that was up to her, but she should prepare a box of raw vegetables for herself instead. Cassie duly cut up carrots, celery, cucumber and cherry tomatoes, and took them with her in a plastic box. Yes, you guessed it: *the children* ate all the raw veggies – admittedly followed by the chocolate – but who knows? If Cassie accidentally 'forgot' to take chocolate and took only apples or vegetables, how much healthier they would all be.

When encouraging your child to eat healthily, remember the benefits of positive reinforcement. Remarks like

'Hey, you polished off those carrots in the fridge pretty quickly – I'll get some more' work better than 'Put that biscuit down and have a carrot instead'.

It might make you unpopular occasionally if you don't give in to their every demand. So? You are a parent, and while they are not paying rent, they abide by your rules, whether it's to do with their food or their behaviour. Your children don't have to like you all the time. They may sulk for a while – but they will just have to get over it. As a parent it is your job to get them to adulthood as healthily as possible. After that it is up to them.

In order to introduce your children to a wide variety of foods, do take them to restaurants. Again, decide what you are going to eat before you go so that you stay calm and in control during the outing – even when you hear yourself snapping, 'Don't do that with your fork.' 'Stop kicking the chair.' 'Mind – you'll spill it.' 'You don't need a straw.' 'For God's sake use a tissue!' – and that's only to your husband.

Encourage your children to take an interest in their own food and learn to prepare it. You could even let them prepare *your* food. Imagine lying in bed one Sunday morning eavesdropping on your dear little offspring happily assisting each other to get your breakfast tray ready: 'Mummy said *I* could do that!' 'She did *not*.' 'You're a liar!' (A crash – crockery breaking. Silence.) 'I'm *telling*!' 'Get the cat's paw out of the bowl, Mum's got to *eat* that.'

Experts agree that most childhood obesity is the result of underactivity rather than overeating, so it's up to you to encourage and, if necessary, participate in any sport that interests them – swimming, tennis, roller-blading.

Spending time with small children can be emotionally exhausting, so I can understand any woman who had even the semblance of a career before motherhood longing to go back to the structure of a day job. Having brought up five children and emerged reasonably sane, may I offer one last piece of advice: never lend your car keys to anyone you gave birth to.

Dealing with Your Mother

Young children growing up are mostly influenced by the same-sex parent: boys by their father and girls by their mother. As the young girl grows up, her relationship with her mother often becomes fraught, and this can continue into adulthood. Ideally, as childhood ends the daughter should separate from her mother psychologically and move on to a mature relationship in which they can communicate with each other as adults and friends.

Sadly, this doesn't seem to happen in real life. Many of my clients have told me the opposite: how childlike they feel in the presence of their mother, as though their relationship is stuck in time. 'I don't know what it is,' sighed one, 'but whatever my mother says, I can't stop myself saying the exact opposite, whether I believe it or not. It's as though I am determined to make her wrong.'

This is not always the daughter's fault. Sometimes it's the mother who simply won't accept that her child is an adult and entitled to lead her own life. A few years ago I was at a family wedding and went to have a word with my mother. She was chatting with an elderly aunt, with whom I had exchanged greetings earlier in the evening. I started to tell my mother something but she interrupted to indicate her companion and say to me, 'Have you said hello to Auntie Renee?' I was 47 at the time – not six!

Clients with a food problem always seem to have mothers who were – and still are – ultra-critical of everything they do, who withhold praise and find fault with every little thing. 'When I was young, whatever I achieved was never enough,' said another client. 'At school, even if I got an "A" for an English essay, my mother would say, "Well it's not very nice writing is it?"' Is it frustration then, or just familiarity, that leads to bouts of overeating whenever these clients return to their family home on a visit? Somehow they can't resist the food their mother prepares for them. The old familiar aromas and tastes still exert a tremendous pull and they eat everything in sight. As one client sighed, 'My mother always told me I had to clear my plate. Now whenever I hear the words "starving children", I start to salivate!'

> You don't need to eat everything that's put in front of you.

A lot of mothers play the guilt card with their adult daughters by interfering in the way they raise their children and complaining that they don't phone or call round to see them often enough. It is as though these mothers are trying to force their daughters to love them out of a sense of obligation. Sadly the only effect it has is to make these daughters exasperated and eager to escape from the constant complaining. 'Whenever I come home from seeing my mother, I eat the entire contents of the fridge!' is a recurring sentiment from my clients.

The only way to deal with this is to manage it. Your mother is not going to change. No matter how difficult you find her, it is important to remember that it is not her behaviour that is causing you distress, but the way you feel and react to her behaviour.

You are an adult now, and even though you may love your mother very much, you have to reconcile yourself to the fact that she just doesn't understand your emotional needs. So? Maybe it's a generational thing: maybe your mother assumed that you didn't need praise because you 'knew' that she loved you and was proud of you. Whatever the cause, you need to break free of the emotional bond and learn not to react to the things she says. Your mother doesn't make you overeat – you do. If she says something outlandish like 'You're too thin – you don't eat enough meat', don't explode and tell her to mind her own business. Just say 'You are probably right' and change the subject. What difference does it make? Don't hand over your power to your mother and let her be the catalyst for a binge.

Dealing with Fear

Many of the women I meet are anxious and fearful about – well, they don't really know what about. They read in the newspaper about some child being abducted, or HRT causing an increased risk of breast cancer and unconsciously experience a flutter of panic. An ambulance wails by and they immediately get pictures in their mind of a loved one tangled in a car wreck. This sort of thinking is prevalent in my post-menopausal clients and it can lead to stressful eating. Food brings instant calmness and blots out the mental turmoil. It is later, when the results of these eating binges become apparent, that anxiety turns into depression. Each client thinks she is the only one who suffers from this and gets embarrassed admitting it.

I assure them that this way of thinking is very common. It is important for them to find someone to whom they can articulate exactly what is worrying them, without interruption or thoughtless interpretations. They need to validate their experience. This often allows them to become detached from their fears and see them for what they are: simply thoughts they have put into their heads which have no basis in reality.

This is harder to do when you have to confront illness and possibly the death of someone close to you, but sometimes it is not our job to question what or why; it's our job to accept what is. Accept what you have instead of questioning what happens to other people.

Some of my younger clients use the fact they are fat as an excuse not to try and achieve anything worthwhile with their lives. 'Who would want to employ me look-ing like this?' The fear of failure is so great that they put up a 'wall of weight' and hide behind that wall. Using food in this way makes them feel safe, as though they have zipped themselves into a fat suit to protect them from the world.

These clients are afraid that if they lost the weight and still didn't succeed, they would no longer have an excuse. Well, if you don't try, you can't fail. I know that if you come out from behind that wall, you have to face the world looking as you do, and other people's comments can be hurtful. But it's not exactly pain-free behind the wall either, is it? Maybe it is time to tackle that weight problem once and for all. You may want to think about this.

Dealing with Forward-projection Anxiety

If you have always turned to food in stressful situations, you can talk yourself into a binge before anything actu-ally happens.

Case Study

Karen was an aerobics teacher whose toned body belied an obsession with food and weight. She told me that she was always either starving or bingeing. With my help, she managed to get into a sensible eating pattern she could live with comfortably on a day-to-day basis. Karen lived with her boyfriend in London and went home to her parents' house in Leeds for an extended stay at Christmas. Much as she loved her mother, Karen was overwhelmed by the thought of all the food she would be surrounded with for two weeks. Karen gravitated towards junk food around 21 December on the premise that 'I'll have to eat all that stuff anyway when I go up north, so I might as well start now and begin eating sensibly again on 1 January' (usually 10 pounds heavier).

Karen was projecting her anxiety to the future and convincing herself that she couldn't cope with something that hadn't even happened. Once she realized what she was doing, Karen was able to form a plan to deal with Christmas. She gave herself permission to eat specific fattening foods, such as brandy butter and Christmas pudding on Christmas Day, and would plan each day's food intake carefully for the rest of her stay. In this way, she stayed in control and did not sink into her usual compulsive eating and subsequent depression.

Case Study

Another client, Sarah, was married for the second time, and both she and her husband had two grown-up children. Sarah got on very well with her step-daughter but her step-son resented the fact she had moved into his family home, and he moved out. His coldness towards her stopped just short of rudeness, all the time.

Understandably, Sarah got very upset at this, and whenever he came round she always ended up bingeing on vast quantities of food to quell the shaky feeling in her stomach. It got to the point that even anticipating a visit could send her running to the biscuit tin. Like Karen, Sarah was projecting her anxiety forward and stuffing herself with food before the guy had even stepped into the house.

My comment of 'You don't even like this man. Why are you letting him make you fat?' seemed to strike a chord with her. Sarah realized she was handing over her control power to someone else, and allowing him to keep her fat. Sarah took back control and was able to stop bingeing in stressful situations.

Dealing with Guilt

Let's look at another couple of examples of how people used food to assuage their feelings.

Case Study

Claire felt guilty because of the feelings of dislike she harboured towards her much older sister, Elise. They had never really got on, even as children, and Claire's out-of-control eating always coincided with a visit to or from her sister, after which she would rebuke herself for her weakness, her shape and her lack of willpower. Instead of defending herself against her sister's snide and sarcastic comments and possibly starting a family row, Claire forced down the angry words with food then shouted at herself for being fat.

I told Claire that it was always easier to feel bad about being fat than it was to face up to the fact that instead of loving her sister, she really didn't like her very much. Once Claire understood that she didn't have to like someone just because she was a close relative, she stopped being affected by her sister's comments.

Case Study

Ginny is another client who was doing extremely well in staying in control of her eating. She phoned me in distress one day because her friend, Roz, had asked her to baby-sit on Friday evening. Ginny had looked after the children before and they loved her. However, Ginny had recently met a rather gorgeous man who had suggested, but not confirmed, going out on Friday night. She told Roz that she 'might have plans for that night'. Roz repeated 'Might have?' in a way that implied she thought Ginny was trying to get out of helping her. Ginny started to say, 'If he hasn't phoned by Wednesday...' but Roz interrupted with, 'It's OK, forget it, I'll ask someone else.' Roz hadn't spoken in an unkind way, but a few minutes later, Ginny found herself picking at some chocolate biscuits.

She knew she wasn't hungry, but couldn't stop eating them. She kept going over the conversation with Roz in her mind, hearing the disappointment and slight disapproval in her voice. It made Ginny anxious just thinking about it. She finished the biscuits then cast around for something else to eat. Instead, she phoned me, saying that she couldn't stop eating and felt fat and horrible.

I told Ginny that she was, in fact, feeding her feeling – the anxiety she felt whenever she had to say 'No' to someone close. But Ginny had translated her feelings into 'fat thoughts' and was only concerned that she 'couldn't stop eating'. Ginny was using her obsession with weight and food to obscure the real issue that sent her scurrying towards the chocolate biscuits. I convinced her that it was OK to say 'No' sometimes and to put herself first without feeling guilty.

Maybe Ginny will continue to have conflicts about what she considers good or bad behaviour. Now that she recognizes that it's not her fat or eating that she feels bad about, she is in a position to work on her real problem, which is her inability to say 'No' comfortably.

Everyone trying to lose weight feels guilty – when they eat something fattening; when they buy chocolate for the family knowing they will end up eating it; when they refuse food someone has prepared for them then go home and binge. Rationalize this: the world didn't come to a shuddering halt because you ate a chocolate brownie. The only promise you have broken is the one you made to yourself. Get over it. Get back on track and move on.

Dealing with 'What If?'

Like Ginny in the example above, one of the reasons you grab for food when you are not hungry is to feed a feeling: whether it's anxiety, apprehension, discomfort or unease. These feelings are vague and manifest themselves as a 'niggle', a fluttering sensation in your stomach that you interpret as hunger and which you attempt to quell by eating something stodgy. The really big emotions like terror, anguish or deep distress take you beyond this 'niggle', and you will often find you are unable to eat in those circumstances.

The fluttery feelings of unease are often the result of the 'what if' thought. 'What if he's had an accident?' 'What if this lump is malignant?' 'What if I lose my job?'

The way to deal with this is to answer the question. Instead of using food to repress the 'what if' thoughts going round your head in some endless loop, take the thought to a conclusion. 'What if he's had an accident?' If he has, you will soon hear about it and will take appropriate action – but you know he's been stuck in meetings before and not realized the time. 'What if this lump is cancer?' Make an appointment with the doctor and get it checked out. It's not 'wasting his time' – that's what he is there for.

You get the idea. If you can put a name to what is causing you discomfort, you can start to look at it with a clear head. All problems require thought and individually tailored solutions. Eating offers precisely the opposite. It inhibits thought and pushes the problem away – only for it to return later. If you are going to ask yourself 'what if?', keep going until you get to the answer. Then you won't need to solve it with food.

Dealing with Comfort Eating

This is important so I hope you get this. All of the above examples can be classified as comfort eating. What you are doing is dealing with all your physical and emotional needs with food. When you don't feel well, you think you need some sugar to give you energy, to make you feel stronger: you are attempting to heal yourself with food. When you are upset, you think you deserve some chocolate to blot out the hurt and make you feel better: you are comforting yourself with food.

You have one fix for everything: getting high with sugar. Emotional hunger feels the same as physical hunger so you are using food as a drug to change the way you feel. Food is your coping mechanism, your best friend. Food never judges you, never rejects you and is always there for you. The fear is always there that if you give up your coping tool you will have nothing left to deal with your problems.

Women in particular are so hard on themselves where the shape of their bodies is concerned. You call yourself names and tell yourself how awful you look because you think this will motivate you to do something about it. Well, that's not exactly working, is it? You do not need guilt or shame or to stick fat, ugly pictures on your fridge door to humiliate yourself into doing something different. It's as though being overweight makes you such a bad person that you need to be punished, so you have to judge and motivate yourself negatively.

Try a Different Outlook

Every person needs some love and unconditional acceptance in their life. Every person fears rejection. You may be an adult but inside you there are still the vestiges of a vulnerable and slightly unsure child who, on occasion, needs someone to put their arms round her and say, reassuringly, 'Don't worry, everything will be all right.' That is why every woman needs three people in her life: a 'mother', a 'friend' and an 'advisor'. You need these three people to be on your side all the time, every minute of every day.

When you are upset and someone has been horrible to you, you want your 'mother'. You want her to comfort you and protect you. Sometimes, as we discussed earlier, your real mother might have got it wrong when you were young. If you told her you were being bullied at school, she might have shrugged it off with, 'Well, you'll just have to learn to stick up for yourself,' instead of comforting you and telling you she would sort it out for you.

Over 90 per cent of the binge eaters I see had a mother who was a perfectionist and constantly disapproved of them when they were struggling to find an identity in the world. Well, you are now an adult, and although events in your childhood undoubtedly shaped the person you are today, it is time to let go of your real mother and become your own 'mother'. What would you *like* your mother to say in the situation you find yourself in? Wouldn't it be something along the lines of

'Never mind, darling, you know your boss can be a total prat sometimes, just ignore it. I think you are doing really well.' Maybe you would feel stupid saying something like that to yourself – but, hey, so what? You are not going to speak out loud, and it would make a change from the negative way you habitually talk to yourself.

There are some things you can't share with your mother but your best friend is always there to take your side, even if you are in the wrong. Would your friend say to you, 'You are such a pig – why did you eat the entire carton of ice cream? You look fat and disgusting'? Of course not. Your friend would say, 'OK, you screwed up. It's done. How could you have prevented that? What should you have done instead? Shoved it in the bin and walked away. So that's what you'll do next time. Don't ruin the whole day worrying about it. Go back to sensible eating and you'll be fine. You've done so well up to now.' Isn't that what you would like your friend to say? Then be your friend – you say it. Tell yourself, 'You look great in those trousers. OK, still a bit of a tummy there but we're working on that.' When faced with a tricky situation say, 'Come on – you can *do* this. You've coped before so you can cope now.'

You also need an advisor/father-figure you can turn to for important decisions. Not for the big stuff like buying a new car or moving to a different area, but the small things that fall into the 'What shall I do about this?' category. Again, your real father may have failed you in this regard when you were young by becoming critical of your choices or exasperated by your behaviour, or simply not being around much, but your personal 'advisor' is always there for you. He wouldn't say things like, 'Oh, for God's sake, why are you so stupid? Can't you even make a simple decision? You are going round in circles.' He would say, 'OK, don't panic. Write down the pros and cons, and make the best choice according to the knowledge that you have. Maybe you need professional help with this before signing anything? Just stay calm. Everything will be all right.' Wouldn't you want someone to give you that reassurance – to say to you, 'Well done, you handled that really well'? Then do it. Be your own advisor.

If you do all of these things, if you are all of these people to yourself, you won't need to comfort yourself with food. I hope that makes sense. The most important relationship in your life is the one you have with yourself. **Get this: sometimes you have to give yourself what you wish you could get from someone else.** You are with yourself 24 hours a day, seven days a week. Would you choose to be with someone who puts you down and says horrible things to you? Of course not. Make your inner voice positive, supporting, uplifting and encouraging. Always be there for you.

You know how you have behaved or responded in the past to particular situations. The challenge now is to stop that past behaviour determining what you will do in the future. If you have binged in response to stress, you are likely to continue doing so unless you have a strategy to deal with it. Work out something that is relevant to you, personally, and stick with it. Reinforce the strategies that work for you, such as never having to eat to please anyone else. You never have to give away your control to anyone else, be it a traffic warden or a close family member. Don't let them be the stress that makes you binge. You are in control of your eating – and your life.

To live like a slim person takes effort, dedication and perseverance for the first six weeks. After that, everything seems to fall into place and it becomes easy. Once you decide you are not going to be fat any more, all you need to do is eat healthy food and practise the strategies outlined in this chapter. The rest will take care of itself.

Telephone Conversation with Client

Three weeks ago Natalie weighed 14 stone 10 pounds.
She made the commitment to stop eating sugar and now
weighs just under 14 stone.

Me: *Hi Nat, how did you get on today?*

Nat: *Er, slight disaster.*

Me: *What sort of a disaster? Weren't you going to something
at your daughter's school this morning?*

Nat: *Yes, it was the summer fête. I was just chatting to a friend
when this lady came round with a tray of fairy cakes and
I absent-mindedly bought one for me and one for the
baby and ate them both. Then I thought, 'Oh God, I was
doing so well, why did I do that?'*

Me: *And God replied…?*

Nat: *Actually, he didn't.*

Me: *Were you hungry?*

Nat: *No, I'd had breakfast. But I thought, well, you know –
it was for charity.*

Me: *No, I don't know. How does that work? Which charity
will benefit from you having a large bum?*

Nat: *It was difficult to refuse actually. The lady was very
persuasive.*

Me: *You mean she grabbed you in an arm-lock and stuffed
the cake into your mouth?*

Nat: *No, don't be stupid. She was very nice.*

Me: *I'm sure she was, but you never have to eat to please anyone else.*

Nat: *Oh come on! Two lousy fairy cakes! Surely that can't do much damage.*

Me: *No, you're absolutely right. Two fairy cakes will not make the slightest bit of difference to a normal person's diet. But you are a binger, Natalie, and once you start eating sugary food – well, you tell me. What happened afterwards? Did you have your planned chicken salad for lunch?*

Nat: *Not exactly. Somehow I didn't fancy it, so I had five slices of toast and butter with melted cheese on top. Then I had the rest of Jake's ice cream. Damn – I've blown it, haven't I?*

Me: *No, of course not. Learning to live like a slim person is not a contest to be completed within a certain time frame. You are bound to have these blips every now and again. The secret is to stop eating fattening food now and get back on track. Don't blow the rest of the day.*

Nat: *(dubious): I'll try.*

Me: *Based on the assumption that every experience is a learning experience, what have you learned from today's events?*

Nat: *That I am a fat, greedy pig?*

Me: *You know what I mean. You have learnt that one taste of sugary food starts you off on a binge, so it's better not to start. How would you handle a similar situation next time?*

Nat: *I guess I should always take a snack with me, like an apple, then if I felt peckish I wouldn't need to go for sugary food if that was all that was available.*

Me: *That's it — you've got it. It's just a matter of planning ahead. Be prepared and you win every time. Tomorrow will be easier.*

Nat: *Yeah — er, I'll just go and chuck out those three chocolate eclairs I bought on the way home then.*

Conversation with Client

C: *Don't ask how I got on — I've had a terrible week. I have not stopped picking and bingeing for five days. I'm so bloated, I feel like a walking water bed!*

Me: *What happened?*

C: *Oh, you know, family stuff. Last year my brother was in financial trouble and I lent him £3,000. He's only paid back £200, and now my sister tells me he and his wife have booked to go on an expensive cruise. I phoned him and he said how dare I discuss his finances with other members of the family. We had a terrible row and he slammed the phone down. Then my snotty sister-in-law came round and called me a lot of names. I told her to get out of my house and, I'm afraid, I sort of pushed her — and now she's saying I assaulted her and…*

Me: *So you are paying her back by getting fat. Makes sense. That'll show her!*

C: *Well, I am just so angry. I lie in bed having furious conversations with them, then I can't sleep and go down and raid the fridge.*

Me: *Do you want to be fat?*

C: *Of course I don't want to be fat! I've lost nearly two stone – and am probably well on the way to putting it back!*

Me: *Then stop now. You have the power to deal with this situation any way you choose – and you don't have to choose food. Understand that this isn't about money. If your brother was desperately ill and needed treatment costing £3,000, you would gladly give it to him. Do you want your brother in your life?*

C: *Of course I do but…*

Me: *Then resolve it. Don't leave it in the hope that it will go away or you will keep having these conversations in your head and get more and more stressed. You want to punish the person who upset you, but the only person you are punishing is yourself. You are handing your power over to your sister-in-law and allowing her to make you fat.*

C: *But she is entirely in the wrong.*

Me: *What does it matter? You can either be right or you can be happy. Resolve it. Contact your brother and talk it through without accusations. Do or say whatever is necessary to arrive at a compromise so you can get your life back on track.*

C: *But she…*

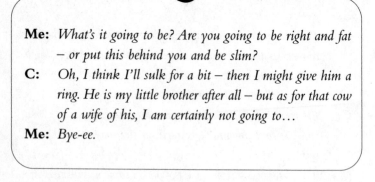

Me: *What's it going to be? Are you going to be right and fat – or put this behind you and be slim?*

C: *Oh, I think I'll sulk for a bit – then I might give him a ring. He is my little brother after all – but as for that cow of a wife of his, I am certainly not going to…*

Me: *Bye-ee.*

Conversation with Client, Sandra, aged 57

S: *I'm really worried about my three grandchildren. I'm sure they don't eat properly. My daughter has a very demanding job and she just gives them ready-made food like fish fingers and tinned spaghetti all the time.*

Me: *How do you know, do you live with them?*

S: *No, but whenever they come and visit they are always holding a bag of crisps or sweets and constantly snacking.*

Me: *Is your daughter fat?*

S: *No she is very slim and belongs to a health club. But I always cooked nourishing meals for my family every day and I expected her to follow my example.*

Me: *Are the children fat?*

S: *No, but I do worry that they aren't getting enough of the proper nutrients. In fact, I recently sent my daughter a newspaper article on the growing trend of childhood obesity.*

Me: *I'm sure she will be eternally grateful for that.*

S: *Funny you should say that because she hasn't actually mentioned it yet. I always give the kids raw carrots when they come to me, hoping she will get the hint. Apart from that, what can I do to ensure they eat properly?*

Me: *Since you are asking my advice, I would say mind your own business. You had your chance to bring up your own children, now allow your daughter and her husband to do the same in their own way. If your daughter is holding down a good job, she must be intelligent, and if the children are healthy and happy, then she must be doing something right. What were you thinking, sending her newspaper articles? You would do well to remember that you are a guest in their marriage and if you continue to make them feel on trial all the time, they will eventually exclude you from their plans. What they need from you is unstinting praise and support, and only give advice if they ask for it.*

S: *Mm, thinking back to when my kids were young, I used to get really irritated when my mother told me what to do…*

Chapter Eight

You've Lost it - Now Keep it Off Forever

🍓 **Don't think about tomorrow. Just do today.** 🍓

I'm sure that at some point in your dieting life you will have stepped on the scales and found that you've reached your desired weight. Ye-e-ss! This is a moment of great joy and you can't believe the excess weight has actually gone. You feel great, you look amazing in your new, smaller clothes and your friends are lavish with their compliments. You realize that you have actually lost the taste for sweet food and have got into the habit of automatically choosing healthy food wherever you go. Even when you see other people eating creamy desserts, you know you would enjoy the taste but have no burning desire to do so – much to your relief. You feel so much better that your commitment to carry on this way is absolute.

Oh yes? I think we have been here before, don't you? So what happened?

Regaining weight you have lost is a depressing, insidious process that seems to creep up on you unawares. It may start with a little slip, when you eat some food you hadn't intended, such as chocolate, or perhaps you felt unable to refuse some home-made cake. Once you got the taste of that, somehow you couldn't stop picking at food for the rest of the day. The next day you resolved to go back on your diet and be 'good'.

However, as the little lapses continued, you found it harder and harder to get back into a healthy eating regime. Gradually, gradually, the weight crept back on again until there you are, gazing miserably at yourself in the mirror and wondering how it all went – literally – pear-shaped. If you are honest with yourself, you will admit that the same patterns have occurred again and again during your life.

You are not alone. Statistics show that only four people out of every hundred keep their weight at the lower level for more than a year. The rest go up and down in a yo-yo spiral, losing and gaining the same, usually 14–20lb (6–9kg), all the time. Although it doesn't sound very much, those few pounds can represent two dress sizes, leading to a wardrobe of 'thin' and 'fat' clothes to match your 'thin' and 'fat' mentality at the time.

Why the Weight Goes Back on

Let's look at some of the main reasons for regaining weight. Does any of the following apply to you?

The Fad Diet

Whether it is the Atkins diet, a 'soup, soup and nothing but the soup' plan, a not-mixing-this-food-with-that diet or cutting out whole categories of food such as wheat and dairy, the fad diet eventually has to come to an end. You can't live for the rest of your life on foul-smelling cabbage soup, or suffer the halitosis of a high-protein diet. All fad diets work the first time you try them, but you can't stay on them forever. Life and 'normal' eating intervene, and though you tell yourself you will go back on your punishing regime next month and lose more weight, somehow you never get beyond day three.

The Occasion Came and Went

You decided to lose weight for a specific event: a wedding, a holiday, a fun occasion like appearing in a charity fashion show. Once that event happened, your motivation dwindled along with the excitement, and you reverted back to the eating patterns that made you fat in the first place.

Christmas

Most people put on a bit of weight during the Christmas break, to the delight of gym owners who gleefully anticipate the profitable rush of new members in January. The seemingly endless round of office parties and family gatherings, followed by New Year parties, can make it incredibly difficult to keep to any sensible eating regime. Plus, of course, there's more alcohol around than usual, which makes it harder to resist the snacks and sweets. So most people give in and accept the inevitable, assuming that the

extra pounds will disappear during January, which they do
– for most people.

If, however, you are a long-haul dieter and prone to
bingeing, the good habits you have carefully built up over
the preceding months can be discarded overnight as you
hear yourself making the old excuses – 'It's cold', 'I'm
starving!', 'January is such a miserable month' – for continuing to eat stodgy, fattening food.

Having a Baby

You really meant to eat sensibly all the way through your
pregnancy. You read all the books, started taking folic acid
and staked out the local antenatal classes. But you felt so
sick during the first three months, and the only thing that
would stay down was banana-and-sardine sandwiches.
Then, when the bulge appeared, you thought, 'Oh this is
ridiculous, I'm going to look fat anyway, so I'll just eat
what I want and go on a really strict diet once the baby is
born. Everyone says the extra weight just drops off if you
breast-feed.' Not in your case, Ducky!

Aiming Too Low

You were a size 10 all through your teens and early 20s –
no problem. So why can't you get down there now? You
did three summers ago – for about 20 minutes (whatever
happened to that ra-ra skirt?) – so why are you struggling
now? Answer: because you are not 18 any more – sorry.

Your body shape and metabolism change as the years go by, and if you continue to aim for a lower weight than you can happily sustain, your dieting efforts are doomed to failure.

The Plateau

When you first embark on a weight-loss regime, the pounds usually drop off at a steady rate. At some point – often around the fifth or sixth week – the rate of weight loss slows down and may stop altogether for a while. This is very disheartening, especially if you have stuck rigidly to your set diet, and you begin to entertain thoughts of 'Well, one little chocolate won't hurt, the diet isn't work-ing anyway.' Disaster. When the scales show a minor gain, after all your hard work, you give up in disgust and revert to your three-bags-of-crisps a day habit.

Too Rigid Diet

Any diet that restricts you to bland 'diet' foods, such as cottage cheese and salad, or cuts out huge swathes of any-thing that helps your day along – tea, coffee, carbs, dairy foods – can't work in the long term. The same applies to a set diet devised by someone else where you eat this for breakfast, this for lunch and this for dinner with no deviation. Detox routines, where you are expected to live for 28 days on seeds, nuts, fruit and vegetables, also fall into this 'too rigid' category. Again, it may work the first time, but once you start to eat normally, the weight will go back on, and the thought of going through that initial headachy withdrawal period once more sends you mouth-first into the biscuit tin.

Have you noticed – all detox-addicts have huge bums? The reason for this is that when you put your body through the trauma of a severely restricted food regime, the first thing you lose is water. As there is very little food to use as energy, your body turns to lean muscle tissue because this is easier for your system to break down than stubborn fat. Fat is the last thing to go because your body has been pro-grammed to hold on to the fat for survival purposes.

Obviously you can't remain on your detox diet forev-er so when you start to eat normally again, the first thing that is replaced is the fat – not the lean muscle. Therefore, every time you go on a severe diet and put the weight on again, you get fatter and fatter. Worse, because your mus-cle mass is now depleted, you don't burn up calories like you used to, so your body will continue to store fat. That is why detox devotees look so flabby. Good game!

My wise guru, Professor John Yudkin, once said to me, 'If anyone mentions the word "detox" in relation to weight loss, you can safely disregard anything further they have to say on the subject.' This was borne out by a recent study of all the popular diets carried out by the *Daily Mirror*'s *M* magazine, where they tested the total fat percentage of the volunteers both before and after the various diets. The only diet that recorded nought per cent fat loss was Carol Vorderman's Detox Diet. No sur-prises there then.

Regular Patterns of Eating Disrupted

Long-awaited holidays, visits to family overseas, having friends to stay for weeks at a time: anything that disrupts your normal daily routine can send you spinning off the rails as far as your diet is concerned. Eating in restaurants night after night, where you have less control over the fat content of your food and you might succumb to tempting desserts, can cause your weight to soar. You miss your weekly body conditioning class or visits to the gym, which gave you a feeling of body awareness and strengthened your dieting resolve. Although you are determined to 'get back to normal' as soon as you get home or the visitors depart, it just doesn't seem to happen.

Addicted to Dieting

You love being on a diet. You devour all the new diet books, it is your favourite subject with friends, you love spouting all the new theories, and you spend most of the day thinking about what to eat and what not to eat. The near-addictive behaviour of serial-dieters suggests that it is the pursuit rather than the attainment of the goal which is the unacknowledged primacy. This sort of dieter delights in lurching from one regime to another, just as the religiously deluded flit from one sect to the next, searching yet never finding. Subconsciously, these dieters don't really want to lose weight for that would mean an end to the search – and then what would they talk about?

Changed Circumstances

An unexpected change to your routine can play havoc with your eating patterns. Whether it's a new job, financial difficulties, perhaps suddenly having to adjust your life to care for a sick relative, there are many circumstances that can affect your plans. As a result, you find yourself grabbing ready-made snacks rather than nutritious meals and snacking on choc-bars instead of your usual fruit. Once you lose the pattern of structured mealtimes, it is very difficult to discipline yourself to eat sensibly.

Stopped Exercising

For some reason – perhaps you were ill or you had to put in extra hours at work – you stopped going to the gym. You were too tired, too busy or couldn't be bothered to change into workout gear, and gradually you lost that energizing 'high' that a session of exercise gave you. Consequently, your muscles got flabby and the weight crept on, giving you another excuse not to go – 'I can't appear looking like this. I'll go back when I've lost a bit of weight.' That vicious circle starts up again.

Unhappy Being Slim

Case Study

Maggie was a plump child whose mother kept telling her how much prettier she would look if she were slimmer. Maggie, wishing to be accepted and loved however she looked, ate out of defiance and grew into a fat teenager and then an even fatter adult. Maggie weighed 14 stone 5 pounds when she first came to see me. After completing my six-week living slim course, she had lost 12 pounds. She sent regular e-mails charting her progress and a Christmas card nine months later saying she now weighed just under 10 stone, had been promoted to head of her department at work and felt great. Three months later, however, she had put back a stone. What happened?

'People treated me differently and I couldn't handle it,' she confessed. 'My bosses seemed to expect much more of me and my colleagues resented my promotion, and the fact that I dressed more smartly and had a new car. I overheard one of them say, "Stuck-up cow – her ego is growing in inverse proportion to her bum," and that hurt. It seemed like it was easier when I was fat.'

Maybe, since Maggie was unsure how to behave as a newly slim person, she came across as conceited and standoffish in her new, expensive clothes, and her colleagues couldn't relate to her in the same way as the 'Fat Mags' they once knew. I advised Maggie to see a therapist friend of mine to learn how to modify her behaviour as a slim person rather than put all that unhealthy weight back on again.

Back to Old Habits

Happily, most people don't have the sort of trauma that Maggie endured and can simply enjoy all the benefits of being slim. The main reason the weight goes back on after a successful diet is that you become complacent. You get used to seeing a slim outline reflected in the mirror. Your friends no longer remark on your achievement. Having successfully stayed off junk food for months, you consider yourself 'cured' of your old bingeing habit. You now seriously think that you can eat whatever you like and the weight will stay off.

Wrong! All the memories of the pleasurable sensation you got from eating sweet, fatty food are stored in your brain – and will come flooding back when you gradually revert to your old way of eating. You forget how wretched you felt when you were fat and lumpy and only remember the succulent taste of toffee-filled chocolate bars or the creamy sensation of Nigella's amazing chocolate-lime cheesecake melting in your mouth. You think you can control it and just have the occasional treat but, to your horror, the scales creep up and up until you are totally out of control once again.

Regaining weight is undoubtedly depressing. But it is important to confront this issue so that you can deal with it effectively and get back on track as soon as possible. Take an honest look back at your life and admit where you went wrong before. Every time you fail at a dieting attempt, it reinforces your victim mentality. You tell yourself that you have 'no willpower' or you can 'never stick to a diet', and these thoughts pull you down and make you feel thoroughly miserable. Your mind even turns to detox and Slimfast.

Everyone goes through difficult and emotional times but the outcome will be the same whether you are fat or slim. The difference between a winner and a victim is being able to get back on track after adversity. A winner is someone who realizes she has allowed her eating habits to go haywire and reaches a point where she is determined to stop and change her life around.

Be honest with yourself. Be a winner, not a victim. That fat didn't just reappear of its own accord. You put it there. It is important to accept this fact so that you can make it different this time.

You might decide that you want to give my method a try. The eating plan seems fairly easy to follow – no sugar, just eat carbs for breakfast and last thing at night – or not – no problem there. Protein at every meal – OK, you can do that. What else was there? Each day for the next two weeks, plan ahead and write down what you are going to eat. Can't be bothered with that. Drink water before each meal. What's the point? Exercise? No time at the moment – tight schedule – deadlines – short-staffed – maybe after Easter. And I'm not quite sure what she means by 'change your inner voice'. What inner voice?

THAT INNER VOICE!! The words and thoughts that have kept you fat all these years. The half-hearted attempts at losing weight without planning, without strategies and without any thought other than getting that weight off as quickly as possible, so that you can go back to 'normal' eating.

The First Three Weeks

If you really want to do this, then listen to me because I am telling you what works. You have tried many diets before and none of them has worked on a long-term basis. Now you know you cannot eat all the fattening food you want and still be slim. That is reality. This time you are not on a diet. Living like a slim person is a philosophy in which you – not food – are in control. It takes time to adjust to any new regime, and if you don't follow it exactly for the first three weeks, the changes – both mental and physiological – won't happen. It takes 21 consecutive days to get the sugar residue out of your system and for your body to make the transition from storing fat to burning fat.

To achieve this, you have to *cut out all foods containing refined sugar.* I hope that is clear. If you eat sugary foods during the first three weeks, you screw up the effect you are trying to achieve. To facilitate these changes you need to eat protein at each meal to promote the release of the hormone, glucagon, which lowers the amount of insulin circulating in the bloodstream. You also need to eat something, however small, every three hours to keep your blood sugar level balanced and to prevent you getting hungry. This takes planning and organization to make sure you have the correct foods at hand in the fridge, the freezer or in your bag.

It also takes three weeks to get your mind accustomed to thinking ahead and gradually changing the way you think about food. All your previous diets have been restrictive – in other words, you have been trying *not* to eat. This time, it simply comes down to choice. You know you can eat whatever you like but you are *choosing* not to eat sugary foods because you know they are bad for your health. The words 'I mustn't' or 'I shouldn't' don't come into this equation. You just don't – end of story. Get off the diet mentality. It takes time to change your mind-set from 'deprivation' to 'freedom', but indeed, having eliminated the cause of your bingeing and extra pounds, you are now free to eat everything else. This is truly liberating. Be happy about this decision.

You may not lose much weight during these first three weeks. Some people do, but those clients over the age of 50 take longer to kick-start the steady weight-loss of one pound a week that we are aiming for. You may react with disappointment at this because you reckon a weight-loss regime should produce instant results. Well, this time you may have to be satisfied with lasting results – which is surely better.

Keep a Food Diary (Just do it - OK?)

When you first start this eating plan, your motivation should be high. If you are to stay the course, however, it is important to get the new habits fixed firmly into your head. Please write down what you are going to eat each day before the day actually starts. Don't skip this bit, however annoying it is to do. New clients are often remarkably unenthusiastic about keeping a food diary, primarily, they say, because they don't have time. If this is your attitude, examine it for a moment. What are you implying here? You have as much time in your day as anyone else; and you devote that time to all sorts of other things. Don't you write a daily list of things that need to be done in your diary or on a notepad? What is so different about a food diary? The answer is often that the food diary benefits no-one but yourself – in which case the unspoken subtext of 'I haven't got time' is 'I haven't got time to spend on myself' or, by implication, 'I'm not worth spending time on'.

If this is how you feel, it may well be contributing to your weight problems so it is worth trying to modify this attitude before you go any further. No-one is more impor-tant than you because if you don't take good care of your-self, how can you look after the people who rely on you? Keep the food diary for the first two weeks. You need to get into the habit of planning ahead for your day so that you don't suddenly look up and realize it is time for a meal and you haven't a clue what you are going to eat.

Once this eating plan is firmly established as part of your lifestyle, you will automatically make the correct choices. At the beginning, though, you need to think this through beforehand in case you have to take something out of the freezer to defrost, or prepare a snack to take with you. Don't wait until you are actually about to eat the food before writing it down. It has to be done the previous evening or first thing in the morning.

Write down exactly what you are going to eat – not just 'protein and salad'. Make it something like 'Afternoon snack: 2 celery sticks stuffed with low-fat cream cheese, 4 large dates. Dinner: chicken breast with broccoli, carrots and baked sweet potato.' Do include snacks and jot down a 'possible extra' such as a glass of wine with a friend after work. *You* are planning your menu, so that *you* are accountable for what you eat. If some item of food isn't written down for that day, you don't eat it.

All this sounds as though you have to become obsessed with food. Not so. It is only until you get used to doing this and it becomes automatic to wake up and think, 'Now where will I be today? Shall I take a snack in the car in case I'm stuck in traffic?'

Planning ahead in this way makes the difference between success and failure. It is easy to stick to a healthy-eating plan when you feel like it. It is when you don't – when you are tired and stressed – that you need to keep going. That is where the planning comes in. If you have a definite plan and activate that plan without letting yourself be sidetracked, you will succeed.

Up until now you have been eating haphazardly, snacking on whatever is available. Now you are in control of your eating and making the right choices to live like a slim person.

Eat Every Three Hours

You also need to make sure you eat every three hours by glancing at the clock when you have finished eating. Check the next meal/snack time, and mentally review what you will be eating. In this way, you look forward to your next meal and it eliminates the urge to cram everything in now. You will find you are perfectly satisfied with your small meals and snacks because you know you are going to have something else soon.

If you find you *are* hungry a little while after eating, check what you last ate. Did it contain enough protein? Did it have a satisfying taste? Did you eat slowly? If so, tell yourself you will have something in half an hour – look at the clock, make it a definite time – then get stuck into some activity that needs your full concentration. After 30 minutes, see how you feel. You may find you are now able to postpone it for another hour. You are not denying your hunger or fighting it, just putting off the moment of indulging it.

Beware of the Sugar-trap

Do not underestimate the power of the sugar-drug to pull you in again. Cravings do not cause physical pain, more a nagging ache as though there is a black hole inside you that needs to be filled – which you interpret as hunger. The difference here is that your body might need food but it doesn't need sugary food. With the right frame of mind, these actual hunger cravings are overcome and will disappear very quickly.

More difficult is the psychological craving, the habitual triggers that have pulled you in before: your mum's home baking, your children's half-eaten dessert, your teatime 'treat'. If you have got into certain habits or rituals, these cause an association of ideas, such as 'I can't have a cup of tea without a biscuit'. During the first three weeks, these triggers or habits may materialize at certain times. By being aware of these high-risk times, you can plan a strategy to deal with them.

It is essential to keep the correct mind-set. If you feel you are making a sacrifice or depriving yourself by giving up sugar, you will fall into the sugar-trap. If you believe that you can eat anything you like but are choosing not to eat sugar because it is detrimental to your health, you will find it easy.

But you must counter the brainwashing immediately before the 'I must eat that' thought takes hold by employing your prepared strategy. Get it into your head: you do not need sugar and you are only torturing yourself by regarding it as a daily treat. It doesn't calm you down, it doesn't make you feel good and the effect is only detrimental. Your body has no use for sugar; therefore it does not really crave sugar. Any craving you feel is only in your head. Whether your craving is the result of a physiological hunger or a habitual trigger, accept it for what it is: a feeling that will soon go away.

Don't be miserable because you have decided not to have dessert at a restaurant. Don't let the thought be 'I want it but I can't have it.' Think instead, 'Ugh, I don't even want that fatty sugary rubbish inside my body.' Eat enough of the starter and main course so that you are pleasantly full and just order coffee. Desserts don't make a meal – they make you fat.

A danger time is when you can't sleep. You are tossing around watching the minutes tick resolutely on, unable to silence the jabbering of your mind, and you just *know* that the answer lies in the fridge. What do you do? Is it all right to go down and eat something? Of course it is – but make sure it is a predetermined choice. If you wander down and start picking, you may start with something innocuous like rice cakes and sugar-free jam, but this won't satisfy you and you will end up going through the biscuit tin. It would be better to have a bowl of cereal with milk, sweetened with Canderel/Equal or fructose if necessary. This will fill you up, calm you down and send you peacefully off to sleep.

Get Active

It is vital to fit in the exercise time so that you increase and maintain your muscle density. You want to lose fat, and if you don't do some form of regular exercise your body will start to break down muscle instead. You may look slimmer but you will still give the impression of being flabby instead of firm and toned. However busy you are, schedule that 15-minute power walk into your day at some point, in addition to a proper workout at least twice a week.

The Days Go By

After about three weeks, you will experience a surge of
energy and be feeling lighter and fitter. You will find your
eating schedule has started to form a pattern and you
don't need to write down what you are going to eat any
more. You just know. You have taken on board some of
the tips, such as having a small snack before you go anywhere, and discover that this really works without spoiling
your enjoyment of a meal later. You are gradually developing your own 'eating blueprint', encompassing the food
you enjoy eating, and repeat this day by day.

Resisting Temptation

The only cloud to mar your progress might be the occasional craving you feel when seeing other people eating
some of your favourite sugary food. Look at the person
who is stuffing in that delicious-looking chunk of
chocolate cake. I bet she is fat. Is that the shape you want
to be? It is very rare to see a slim person eating that type
of synthetic-looking stuff, for slim people would rather
be slim than eat junk. In times of temptation, check out
the following:

★ You think it would make you happy? Wrong.
★ You would enjoy the taste? You would probably be
   disappointed.
★ How would you feel afterwards? Bloated – and you'll wish
   you hadn't eaten it.

You may be envying that person, but even as she's eating it she is wishing she wasn't, and she is envying you because you're not. Wouldn't you love to ask her, 'Why are you eating that? Do you want to be fat?' and see what she says?

Stop envying people who say they can 'eat whatever they like'. If they are slim, 'what they like' is healthy food. If they are fat, who needs it? These people would love to be slim but they are hooked on sugar and don't know how to break free. But you do. Immediately employ your phrase 'Don't take the first bite' – or whatever – and remind yourself how much better you feel now. Remove yourself from the sight of the food as soon as possible and the feeling will pass. Allow your 'friend' to tell you 'Well done, that was a bit tricky but you handled it very well.'

Staying Positive

You need to keep up this encouraging attitude at all times. Your thoughts will determine whether you win or lose. Do not allow yourself to either think or talk about any real or imagined pleasure you used to get from eating certain foods. Switch it immediately to remembering the feelings of bloatedness, misery and remorse that always followed an eating binge.

Wipe out negative thoughts such as 'I am so tired, I can't do this' as soon as they appear. I know you can't 'stop' a thought popping into your mind, but you can consciously substitute a new thought before the physiological effects connected with the first thought take hold, such as weakness and imagining you 'need' some sugar. Acknowledge the thought then redirect it along the course you want to go.

We all have memories of past failures and bad times buried in our subconscious. If you dwell on these you can unwittingly make them your current goal. The only way to get rid of a bad feeling is to overlay it with a good feeling. Stop giving power to the past and it will immediately lose its power over you. Do not underestimate yourself. You are strong and capable. Everything you do is your choice, whether it seems that way or not.

The most common cause of negative thoughts that block your efforts to reach your goal is a tendency to exaggerate the difficulty of what you are trying to achieve. For example, thinking 'It will take forever to lose six stone.' You only have to decide how to behave now, this minute. You can't control the future or how you will react at that time. Concentrate on staying in control now, today, rather than focusing on the result. Reinforce your positive affirmations: you are going to have a good day; you feel great.

Rewards and Penalties

You have to be tough on yourself because no-one else is going to be. It may help to instigate a system of rewards and penalties. One of my clients keeps a 'no-sugar calendar'.

She ticks every successful sugar-free day, and when she has accumulated 10 consecutive ticks, she treats herself to a non-food reward – anything from a new lipstick to highlights in her hair. A cross instead of a tick means she has to forego watching an episode of her favourite soap.

In the past, this client always found it difficult to stick to a regular exercise routine. Now she doesn't allow herself to put on her make-up until she has completed her morning walk. This works for her. Do what works for *you*.

The Weeks Go By

One of the things that makes it more difficult to stick to a sensible eating plan is waiting for a result. If you are studying for an exam, you have achieved your objective as soon as you have passed. Waiting for the weight to go is stressful because you have been brainwashed into thinking that if you have been 'good' for a certain number of days, you should be rewarded with a smaller dress size.

If you think, 'I haven't eaten sugar for four weeks now and I've only lost three pounds,' then you are simply waiting to start eating it again. This is the 'what's the point?' mind-set, the 'reward for being good' mind-set. You are prepared to wait a certain amount of time, but if it doesn't happen fast enough for you, you are out of here! Far from feeling free to eat loads of other food, all you are doing is tormenting yourself with thoughts of sugar-laden food. This 'waiting-for-something-to-happen' is a recipe for failure because the cravings will just get more intense until you give in.

But while you are waiting for things to happen, they *are* happening but you are just not conscious of it. If you can stay off sugar, the residue will leave your body, the craving will disappear, and the weight will go, I promise.

Avoid the Scales

So do refrain from weighing yourself every day. The greatest problem I have with clients is stopping them jumping on the scales at every opportunity. It is the over-emphasis on weight-loss that obscures the more relevant issues of constant or compulsive overeating. I can't tell you the number of times a client has said to me, 'I felt really thin and when I put on my jeans they were baggy round the bum. I was so thrilled I just had to weigh myself, and do you know, I hadn't lost a single pound! I was so pissed off, I couldn't get it out of my mind all day and ended up eating two chocolate wafer biscuits at tea time!'

Please be aware of this. 'Living slim' is a continuous process, and the weight-loss is a by-product of this process. If you focus all your attention on the scales, you are allowing a mechanical object to determine whether your mood will be upbeat or downbeat. Do you see that? People don't get upset at what happens; they get upset if something they *expect* to happen doesn't. If I said shut your eyes and I will pop a sweet into your mouth, but instead I gave you a salty olive, you would recoil in surprise. Yet if I had told you I was going to give you something salty, you would have accepted that quite happily.

When your expectation is thwarted, it changes your mind-set and makes you unhappy. This applies in most areas of your life. As one client told me, 'When I got married I saw myself in years to come as a slim yummy-mummy with delightful children. Instead I am this fat 45-year-old lump with a teenage grouch who slams her bedroom door in my face.'

Stay in Control

Be realistic and accept that there is a connection between the food you eat and your weight. Your fat cells never have a day off. Perfectly rational and intelligent people have said to me, 'I've been so good and I cannot believe I have put on a pound this week!' In one case, when I pointed out from my notes that a client had celebrated her birthday with a boozy party and ate everything in sight, she said, 'But that was five days ago. I've been really strict ever since.' Come on now! This is living in a state of denial. Take accountability for your actions. The psychologist Dr Phil McGraw's admonition, 'When you choose the behaviour, you choose the consequences' is so true.

Once you get in control of your eating and your excess weight starts to go, the new self-confidence that emerges will make you much stronger. You will probably discover that you are able to face anxiety and give your problems their proper names. All this happens very gradually of course, but recognizing a problem for what it is will put you in a better position to find a solution that doesn't involve food.

Hitting the Dreaded Plateau

The next possible setback that may hit you takes place a few weeks later. Your weight has been dropping steadily – albeit slowly, but that's OK – and you reach the aforementioned plateau, when for about two weeks you don't lose any weight at all. You are sticking faithfully to your eating blueprint – no sugar, nothing really fattening – but the weight is static.

Be prepared for this: a plateau is simply a barrier you have to break through in order to get where you're going. It is your body doing a sort of mental and physical stock-taking before moving on to the next phase. Don't allow yourself to start thinking, 'It's not working so what's the point?' You have lost water and some fat. Now your body wants time to readjust and sort itself out before releasing any more fat. This pause is also to test your mental resolve to see if you are serious about sticking to a healthy way of eating and not relapsing as you have done in the past.

Reinforce your original motivation. You hated being fat and you are feeling so much better now. Just hang in and keep going day by day. The weight will go and maybe, during this time, your body will take the opportunity to shrink itself down a bit, so even though the scales are static, your waistband will be flapping three inches away from your body.

We are all different. We all lose weight at a different rate. Because you are not restricting your food intake, the weight loss may be slower than you would like. This can be frustrating for chronic dieters who are accustomed to the 'high' that usually follows a weight loss. Please be patient here; you are now watching your eating instead of watching your weight, and the result will be a gradual – occasionally spasmodic – shrinking of your body.

You may also have to go through an exercise 'barrier' before it feels easy and natural to 'jok around the block' without getting puffy and breathless. When you first start exercising after years of inactivity, it may seem desperately hard. Don't give up and start thinking you can't do it. Take the pace down a notch if you feel exhausted – fastwalk instead of trying to increase to a half-walk-half-jog. Suddenly there will be a breakthrough when you will be amazed at how quickly your level of fitness accelerates and how much more energy you have. But you have to persevere to get there.

Audit Your Wardrobe

The next step in your route to living slim is to audit your wardrobe. Why are you still hanging on to all those clothes? How many shapes of 'you' are there in those cupboards? The clothes belonging to compulsive eaters reflect their aspirations, their anguish and their compromises. Most people throw out clothes they haven't worn for the past two years. Compulsive eaters never dare throw anything away. Their past is always their future. The thought is always there that 'Maybe I will fit into this again one day' or 'If I gain weight I'll need this.'

Come on now, it's time for a clear-out. Chuck out anything that doesn't fit *now*. All that should remain are clothes you are happy and comfortable in and that look nice. If there are one or two things you want to keep that are just a bit too tight, then hang them in another room. Opening your cupboard every day and finding clothes that don't fit is a dispiriting experience and a form of daily criticism.

It may be hard for you to let go of the skinny clothes because they represent hope, and the fat clothes because they represent safety. But by the time you have stabilized at the weight you want to be, they will probably all be out of fashion anyway.

Now go and buy some new clothes. Go on, have a good old trying-on session and buy something nice. Don't look at the size. Look at the garment and, if you like it, buy a size that fits, regardless of the number on the label. Sizes vary so much, especially now that so many clothes are imported, and a size number is very much like the number on the scales – it can affect how you feel. Just use your eyes and your body to figure out what you'd like to wear, and remember that the goal is comfort and looking good, no matter what your size.

You no longer need to wear clothes that are tight as a reminder that you should lose weight or in the hope that someday soon it will fit. Dress for now.

Reassessing your wardrobe is all a part of accepting yourself now, as you are – which is the only way to facilitate change. Once you accept yourself as you are, you have a choice about what you want to do. If you have ever said, 'If only I were thinner, I would apply for a better job', you need to evaluate your situation independently of your shape. Do you want to make a move or not? If you do want to but are afraid, what is really standing in your way? Don't allow your weight to determine how you behave. You are entitled to the best things in life, the same as everyone else.

The Months Go By

Once you get into the swing of living slim, it becomes easy. Days blend into weeks, then months, and the food patterns remain constant. But a corner of your mind has to be continuously vigilant, especially on 'down' days. It only takes one puff to get a smoker hooked again. Stay off sugar, whatever else you may eat when you get a niggly feeling. You may have lost some weight but the problem is still there. It doesn't matter what you have for lunch or dinner, it's how you live your life. And it's the same life as you lived before with the same characters re-enacting the same scenarios that caused you to binge in the past. Now you are able to control this – but there may be the odd time when you can't.

Managing a Relapse

☝ **The odd binge is not a sign of failure – it's** ☝
a learning exercise for next time.

You have to recognize that you are a human being and, sooner or later, you will have a slight relapse. The signs to watch out for are irritability; feeling a bit weepy; getting overtired; feeling emotionally fragile, edgy, stressed; being unable to concentrate; feeling inadequate in some way. These are all warning signs of a relapse and you may find yourself back in your kitchen munching through a packet of biscuits.

This is a danger time because that slight slip – biscuits – could so easily turn into a full-scale binge unless you take appropriate action immediately. The thought 'I've done it now' can undermine your whole way of thinking and behaving, and could set the scene for further bingeing. It's too late for 'Don't take the first bite' because you've already done it – so issue a command to yourself: 'STOP EATING NOW!' Say it forcefully and out loud. Get rid of any remaining binge-food. In the bin – *now*. Remove yourself from the kitchen and do something else – anything – that will fully occupy you for the next half-hour until you calm down.

Then have a think. What caused that lapse? What were

you thinking, feeling, picturing just before you grabbed the biscuits? Did something specific happen or was it just a vague sense of unease? Try and give it a name, even if it was just a feeling. Maybe you felt shaky? ('That cyclist didn't have to be so rude, I just didn't see him.') Or perhaps envious? ('Neighbours off on another cruise – am I the only one who works around here?') Or just irritated and fed up? ('I can't believe she still hasn't tidied her bedroom!')

Is there something hanging over you? ('Why can't I just walk in there and ask him for a pay rise?') Is there a problem that needs solving? ('Can we manage without a bank loan?') Whatever it is, if it can be solved, then take the necessary steps to deal with it. Even deciding *not* to deal with it is a decision.

If you practise analysing each situation and putting a name to it whenever you are tempted to indulge in mindless eating, you will soon recognize the warning signs and be able to take evasive action to prevent it happening.

Once you have recovered your composure, remind yourself of how well you have done up to now, how much better you feel. Then determine not to blow all you have achieved over the past weeks. If thoughts of sugary food keep popping into your mind during the next few hours, wipe them out by pressing a mental 'erase' key and substitute positive thoughts of you looking gorgeous in that new dress I told you to buy earlier.

This sort of conscious thinking is the 'remote control' of your subconscious mind to program yourself for success. Watch out if you start thinking phrases like 'I'll start again tomorrow'. This is a tricky one. And the old favourite 'I'll only eat fruit tomorrow' is another way of letting yourself be controlled by food.

Understand that failure is an event, it is not a person and it is not *you*. You can start again. Yesterday ended last night. Today is a brand new day and it's yours.

You do, however, have to be careful on the day after a slight lapse, because old tastes now reactivated can carry on into the following day. Do not attempt to punish yourself by having a 'diet day' if you have eaten something you didn't intend to. It is bound to happen, so just use it as a learning experience to prevent a similar situation arising again, and move on. Stick to your eating blueprint. One fattening snack won't alter the outcome. It is what you eat on a day-by-day basis that determines how you look in the long term. Your greatest strength is resisting the first compulsive bite.

When you work out your own eating plan, it becomes the basis of your food lifestyle, whether you are trying to lose weight or not. It is something that you plan, just for yourself, with the food you enjoy eating and the most appropriate food for your health and wellbeing. Sugary food, you now realize, falls into neither of these categories. Think of your daily eating blueprint as the norm – the eating plan you return to after deliberately sampling some fattening food or returning from holiday or an unplanned mini-binge. This is your day-by-day eating plan by which you now live your life.

Six Months Go By

We've talked before about the danger of getting complacent, especially during the weight-loss phase. Now that
you have settled into your new lifestyle, it's important to
remember the potential pitfalls. If you think you are
'cured' and can have a 'little bit' every now and again,
you will gradually put on weight. It won't happen
immediately, but sugar has an insidious way of creeping
back into your life if you let it. Although you are well
into your new eating plan, as the months go by there is
always the temptation to reward yourself for being
'good' with a little bit of sugary food.

You might start telling yourself you are in control now
and it can't do any harm. Don't do this unless it is a
planned, carefully thought-out occasion. Don't torture
yourself by trying to eat a little bit of a food that triggers
your compulsive eating behaviour. Just like smokers and
alcoholics, you must recognize a substance you can't control. Logically, you should be able to have a little bit without any adverse repercussions, but you can't control sugar
with logic. This food evokes memories, feelings and cravings buried in your subconscious mind, which flood into
your conscious mind and set up a violent craving for more
of the same. Once your taste buds are activated, it's good-
bye to logic, willpower, motivation and good intentions.
No-one puts weight back on deliberately. Those who do
really thought they had beaten their cravings and could
control sugary foods by eating 'just a little'. Trust me, it
doesn't work.

The answer is not to have sugary food in the house. Even though you can safely ignore it most of the time, you know exactly where to go if your control slips. If you could live with these foods around, you wouldn't have had a problem all these years. Don't provide yourself with ready temptation. It's not worth it.

Time will Tell

People who are most successful at losing weight this gradual way are bemused when others exclaim about the weight they've lost. They know that their outline has become narrower, but because they have been looking in the mirror and accepting themselves at each stage, they don't see themselves as looking so radically different.

Accept that there is no hurry and you will eventually reach and stabilize at the weight you were meant to be. You may experience another couple of plateaus when the scales show the same number for a couple of weeks, but your clothes will feel looser. That's fine. If you can stick with your eating plan and exercise regularly, you will get there. All you have to do is choose the right attitude and behaviour to generate the right results. You have to establish a certain positive mind-set that boosts you all the time. This means ditching the deprivation frame of mind and substituting 'freedom'. You are free from the sugar-trap that has made you fat and miserable in the past. That is *good* so be happy that you don't have to eat that stuff any more.

You know that some days will be easier than others. But if you know precisely what you want and what you are aiming for, and accept that there are real consequences for not sticking to your plan, your determination will pay off.

The Years Go By

Once you have stabilized at your desired weight (I repeat *stabilized*) – however long that takes – and are happily living within your chosen eating blueprint, do allow yourself the occasional treat. You can have potatoes or rice with your evening meal now and again. If your weight starts to increase you can always cut them out. Give yourself permission to have a fattening dessert at a party and eat it with enjoyment and no guilt, knowing that you will continue with your normal eating plan the following day. Don't let your rigid 'all-or-nothing' diet mentality rule your life. You are now free – and in control of your eating.

Being 'in Recovery'

However, you should still consider yourself to be a 'recovering binger'. The electro-chemistry of your brain will still kick in the moment you encounter stress and tell you that you need to eat. According to research done at Sydney University in Australia, when cocaine addicts were shown only the instruments for application, they got an urge to use the drug. When these people had a brain scan, the cortex – the area where memory is kept – showed more activity than other areas of the brain. So be vigilant.

Constantly remind yourself why you are doing this: how good you look, how clear your skin is, how much more energy you have. Whatever happens in your life, don't let negative thoughts take hold and pull you down. No-one is immune to this, but you just have to manage it. If I didn't practise what I preach, I would be twelve stone instead of seven-and-a-half.

Dealing with People's Reactions

Don't be embarrassed to refuse food – it's more embarrassing being fat.

Obviously people will notice your weight-loss and their reactions may be varied. Don't be put off by anything anyone says. Some people will say how fantastic you look – others, like your mother or your still-fat friends, will say you are too thin. People resent change. It makes them uncomfortable and unconsciously they want to preserve the status quo. Members of your family may also try to sabotage your efforts by buying your favourite chocolates or saying things like, 'You looked a lot better when your face was just a little fatter.'

So You're Slim - So What?

You should also realize that being slim is not a panacea for all your problems. How often have you said, 'If only I were slim, everything else would just fall into place'? Well, it doesn't quite work out like that. Obviously, being supple and slender and liking yourself gives you much more confidence, but life isn't easy whatever you weigh. You might feel more vulnerable now because you can no longer use your fat as a buffer between you and your feelings, fears and the hurt inflicted by others.

Previously, you could always blame your fat for your disappointments, failures or mistakes, instead of accepting these setbacks realistically and using them as opportunities for growth. Well, that's in the past. It's over, you can't change it. The past only exists in your mind. Move on.

You Always Have a Choice

It may be hard sometimes to stick to a sensible eating plan but it's not as hard as *not* doing it. Continuing to be fat and out of control around food is much harder to live with. Every time you are tempted by fattening food, you have to make a choice. Decide whether you are going to throw the food away or eat it – with the full knowledge that if you do, you are deliberately choosing to be fat. You know what they say: there are no victims, only volunteers. But whatever action you choose, take responsibility for it – don't blame the food or stress or whoever upset you earlier that day. Learning to throw fattening food away is not wasteful; it is an act of self-acceptance. It is more wasteful having three sets of clothes.

As the years go by, you will obviously experience changes and the normal ups and downs of life. Sometimes you may go through a tricky patch that lasts several months, causing your food selection to go haywire. Recognize and accept the fact that your weight may go up a bit from time to time, but in the grand scheme of things, this means nothing. Being aware that this can happen will save you from allowing destructive thoughts and behaviours to take a permanent hold.

You know you can get back on track whenever you choose to do so, simply by deciding on a course of action, starting immediately. Cut out the sugar. Plan ahead and write down what you are going to eat for a week. Whatever happens, don't give up on the exercise. A brisk walk, a body conditioning class, a session in the gym will clear your mind and make all the difference to the way you handle any situation. You are accountable. You are in control of your life. You always have a choice.

So – let's begin. You *know* what to do. I have given you all the tools. All you have to do is use them. Let's have a quick look in the toolbox to start you off:

★ On a day-to-day basis, don't eat obviously fattening food.

★ Eat regularly – watch the clock – don't let more than three hours go by without eating.

★ Plan ahead for your day – flash through your mind

where you will be and what you will eat.
★ Always have plenty of the 'correct' food in the house.
★ Take food with you if you will be away from home for several hours.
★ Have a strategy for dealing with 'trigger situations', such as eating before you go out.
★ Don't seek out your favourite fattening food in shops or at parties. Cravings start with your eyes.
★ Have a phrase ready for moments when you are tempted by your trigger food: 'Don't start, don't get the taste', 'Don't take the first bite', 'You are not a dustbin'.
★ Don't let two days go by without doing some form of exercise.
★ Talk to yourself in a positive way all the time. For example, 'You handled that really well'.
★ Be careful of phrases like 'I'll start again tomorrow'.
★ Learn from slip-ups. Contain binges as soon as possible. Get back on track immediately with your normal eating plan. Do not 'diet' to punish yourself for overeating. It doesn't work.
★ Don't pick - *ever*.
★ Constantly remind yourself why you are doing this. Remember how awful you felt when you were fat and lumpy and your clothes were tight. Feeling slim, positive and liking yourself is more important than eating chocolate.

Absolutely!

Conversation with Client

Lisa, aged 30, has come to the end of a six-week 'Living Slim' course with me, adhering to the principles laid out in this book. This is our final consultation.

Me: *You have done so well, Lisa – 13 pounds in six weeks is pretty good. How do you feel?*

L: *I feel brilliant. All my clothes are loose, I have loads of energy and I never get hungry. I feel confident that I can carry on with this and lose the extra stone. I am really into the 'jok-around-the-block' and feel edgy if I miss it. I also keep a copy of your last book,* Stop Whingeing!, *by my bed to dip into now and again to reinforce the strategies.*

Me: *Actually it's* Stop Bingeing! *but that's great. What was the most helpful thing about the course?*

L: *Learning to plan ahead what I was going to eat each day. I realize now that I've always just picked at food without thinking and wondered why I couldn't lose weight. All that is now in the past – it's over – finished – it's geography –*

Me: *Surely you mean 'history'…?*

L: *Now I mentally whiz through my day, and once I know what I am going to eat and when, I can just relax and get on with it. This has taken all the stress out of eating. Also, having a snack before I go anywhere has been the best tactic for helping me stay in control.*

Me: *What was the hardest thing?*

L: *I thought it would be giving up sugar, but surprisingly that wasn't too difficult, especially as you said I could use fructulose on my cereal.*

Me: *You mean 'fructose'.*

L: *Whatever. Once you explained that losing weight starts in your mind, I decided to try a little mental subterfuge. A few years ago, I was violently ill with food poisoning after eating shellfish and vowed never to touch it again. I decided to equate sugar with shellfish and any craving instantly disappeared.*

Me: *Good thinking. What are your fears for the future?*

L: *At the moment I feel really confident, but that is because you have been phoning me every day. What happens once I have lost the extra weight? Will I put it all back on again like I have done before? Suppose I break the diet and eat something fattening?*

Me: *You can't 'break the diet' because there is no diet to break. You are eating normal food – food that you choose to eat – and the only thing you have cut out is refined sugar. When you have stabilized at the weight you want to be, you may decide that you will eat something sugary and fattening on a particular occasion, but as long as it is a premeditated decision and not an 'Oh sod it' binge decision, it will be fine. You will eat it and enjoy the taste then immediately go back to your personal eating blueprint. Don't be nervous about doing this. It won't be a problem – unless it happens every few days. The most* important thing is not the food you eat, but being in control of the food you eat. Anyway, I'm not leaving the country – you can always phone me if you need to.

L: That's reassuring. The best thing for me about doing this course is that I have stopped my midnight binges. If I couldn't sleep I would sneak down to the kitchen and eat a whole tub of Tom & Jerry's ice cream. I don't do that any more.

Me: It's Ben.

L: What is?

Me: The ice cream. It's Ben & Jerry, you said…

L: Instead I put on some music and sing along until I fall asleep. My favourite track is 'Bridge over Troubled Water' by Simon and Garfinkle.

Me: You mean Simon and – Oh, never mind! Your weight is going so at least you've got that right. You are there, Lisa, well done.

From Me to You

Obviously, my clients are not as dippy as I have made them appear in this book! They are ordinary people, just like you, with careers, families and responsibilities, but have never been able to control their fluctuating weight.

Most people who work with me let go of the concept of dieting, set up their new eating blueprint and break their circuit of addiction within a few weeks. As the months go by they may have the occasional blip but they all lose weight eventually and stabilize at the lower weight.

The initial questions new clients ask are about weight loss: how much will they lose? How long will it take? As they get into it, they develop new measures of progress: how did the day go? How will they handle tomorrow's board meeting when everything stops for coffee and Danish? (Answer: take their own snack for that time.)

For a binger to live comfortably, to know what they are going to eat each day and to have more time free from obsessive thoughts about food and weight are major accomplishments that were formerly unimaginable. In the end the loss of pounds is an added bonus, a side effect of the improved quality of their lives.

For you to achieve permanent weight loss, you have to be totally, consciously aware of yourself and everything you do, think and feel. The things that go right in your life do so because you make them go right. You succeed because you make the right choices and behave in ways to generate the right results.

You can *do* this. I send love and best wishes for your continuing success as a slim person and if you get stuck – well, this book isn't going to disintegrate. You can read it again! Good luck.

The Binger's Prayer

Our God, who art in Bourneville
Cadbury be thy name.
Thy Fruit 'n' Nut, thy Milk Tray
In Tesco, as it is in Selfridges.
Thy choca-mocha latte will be done
As it is in Starbucks.
Give us this day our daily Twix
And forgive us our indulgences
As we forgive them who write diet books.
Lead us not into McDonald's
And deliver us from Pizza Hut.
For mine is the Bounty, the Mars Bar and the Crunchie
In stress and maternity
Now and forever After-Eights
Ah women!

Make
www.thorsonselement.com
your online sanctuary

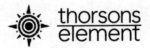